Lived Experiences of People with Recently Diagnosed Multiple Sclerosis

Artwork: Hannah Laycock

Cover: Untitled 12, *Perceiving Identity*, 2015

p. 8, Untitled 09, *Awakenings*, 2015

p. 22, Untitled 16, *Awakenings*, 2015

p. 42, Untitled 14, *Awakenings*, 2015

p. 58, Untitled 06, *Awakenings*, 2015

p. 74, Untitled 08, *Perceiving Identity*, 2015

p. 96, Untitled 04, *Awakenings*, 2015

p. 109, Untitled 09, *Awakenings*, 2015

License HL0013, 22/10/16

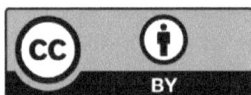

ISBN 978-94-6332-158-7

http://hdl.handle.net/11439/2856

Lived Experiences of People with Recently Diagnosed Multiple Sclerosis

An Analysis Drawing on Phenomenology and Ethics of Care

Geleefde ervaringen van mensen met een recente diagnose Multiple Sclerose

Een analyse aan de hand van fenomenologie en zorgethiek

(met een samenvatting in het Nederlands)

PROEFSCHRIFT

ter verkrijging van de graad van doctor
aan de Universiteit voor Humanistiek te Utrecht
op gezag van de Rector Magnificus prof. dr. Gerty Lensvelt-Mulders
ingevolge het besluit van het College voor Promoties
in het openbaar te verdedigen
op 6 maart 2017 om 12.30 uur

door

Archibald de Ceuninck van Capelle
Geboren op 17 mei 1977 te Dordrecht

Promotores:

prof. dr. Frans Vosman, Universiteit voor Humanistiek

prof. dr. Leo Visser, Universiteit voor Humanistiek

Beoordelingscommissie:

prof. dr. Raymond Hupperts, Maastrichts Universitair Medisch Centrum

prof. dr. Gerty Lensvelt-Mulders, Universiteit voor Humanistiek

prof. dr. Huub Middelkoop, Universiteit Leiden

prof. dr. Stuart J. Murray, Carleton University, Ottawa

prof. dr. Jeannette Pols, Universiteit van Amsterdam

Dit proefschrift werd mede mogelijk gemaakt met financiële steun van het Nationaal MS Fonds. De publicatie van dit proefschrift werd mede mogelijk gemaakt met financiële steun van de Stichting MS Research.

Table of Contents

Discussion

PREFACE

My journey with ethics of care and research started in the winter of 2010/2011. During my work as a health care chaplain I had become, in the decade before, acquainted with the efforts of many clients and patients (mostly elderly, but also younger persons) to come to terms with a sudden and unexpected loss of health and to live with a permanently reduced health condition on a daily basis. Although I and many other care workers I had worked with, were by professional experience familiar with the patients' perspective on illnesses and care, I discovered that it was very difficult for me and others to insert this perspective in interdisciplinary encounters as a durable element of professional care, beyond the categorization as "anecdotal" and of "personal preferences". My doctoral research of the patient perspective on living with recently diagnosed multiple sclerosis (MS) is partly meant as an effort to address this problem. How can the perspectives of patients be properly addressed scientifically and what does that imply for re-categorization in the helping professions? I hope that my thesis about the patient perspective contributes, in the end, to a more solid integration of this perspective in practices of professional care, particularly in care for men and women with MS.

Just like many other projects of research, this dissertation required a lot of solitary work; reading, searching, thinking and writing. The course of the work included detours, excursions, deviations and even dead ends. My wife Margot and our children Kasper, Tamar and Jonas have witnessed year after year how I toiled over my research, often not knowing what occupied my mind, while they watched me working behind my laptop. Their love, patience and support have been invaluable for me. Also I want to address to the men and women with MS who kindly agreed to be interviewed for this study. The conversations with them and some of their partners allowed me to get an exploratory view on the often silent and subtle worlds of sense making that remain frequently out of view in regular practices of efficient, rationalized and economized health care. To these men and women I dedicate this study.

Archie de Ceuninck van Capelle
December 2016

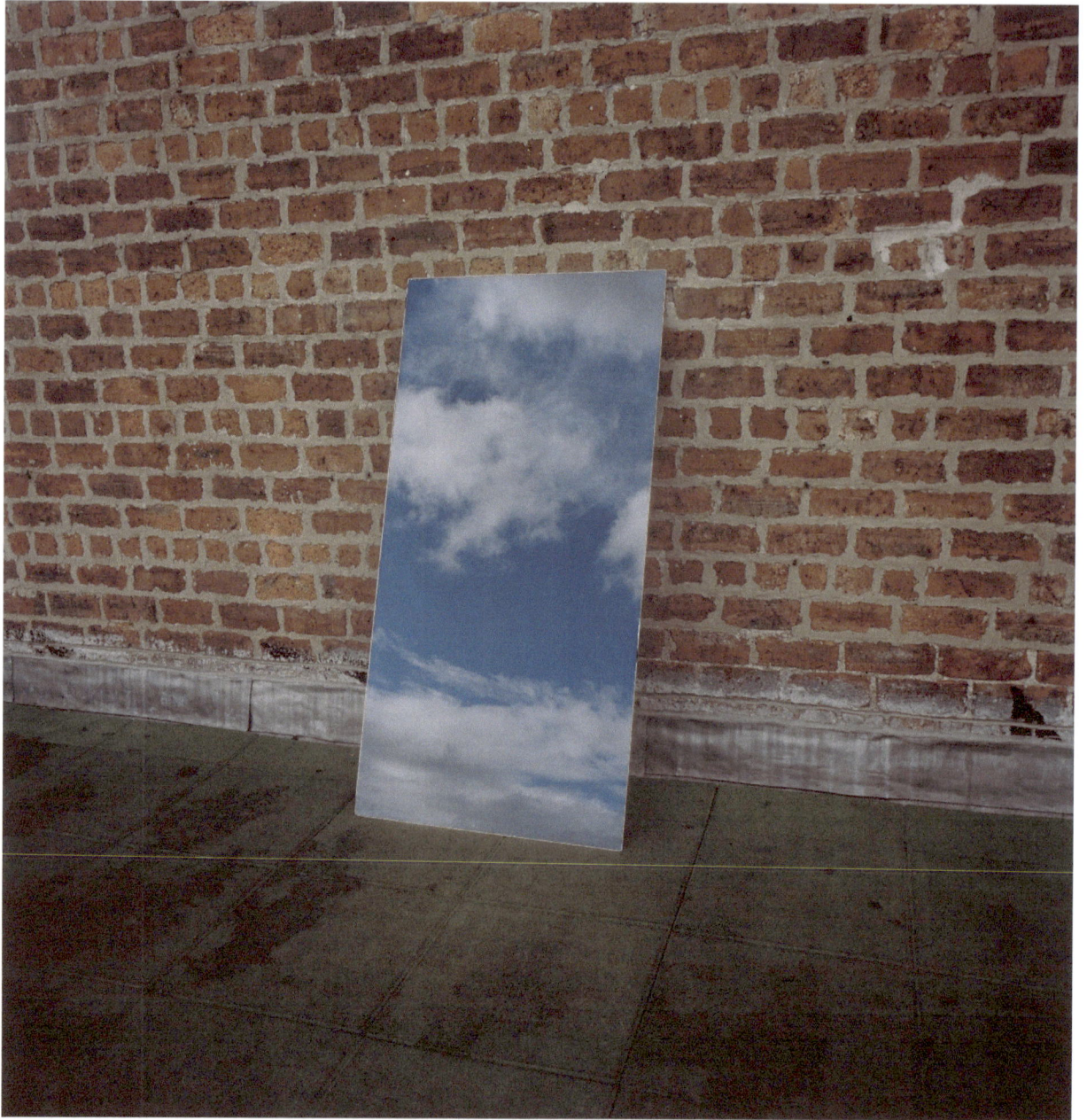

INTRODUCTION

Having stated the goal of this study – contributing to the improvement of care in MS – we outline the basic tenets of the type of phenomenology that constitutes the theoretical framework of our study. We delineate how an ethic of care can be conceived of as a phenomenological approach to a relationship-based and empirically grounded ethics. Next we review extant research on good care (taken as a normative concept) for people with MS. We learn from this review that considerable technical and medical advances in MS care in recent decades have strengthened the position of the creators and owners of specialist technical knowledge. But the "voice of experience" – proper to the patient – seems to have only been weakened. This observation leads to an interpretation of our research question as a mission to retrieve the voice of the patient by 'diving' as deep as possible into the lived experiences of people with MS. The chapter continues with a presentation of the research design drafted to take on this mission. An outline of the study's chapters concludes this introduction.

Improving professional care for people recently diagnosed with MS

These days the improvement of professional care is at the top of the agenda for every stakeholder in professional healthcare: patient organizations, physicians, employers, insurance companies, pharmaceutical companies and governments. Programs for improvement of professional care are multifarious. An example of such a program was "Menslievende Zorg" (MLZ) [Professional Loving Care]. This five-year program (Baart, Vosman et al., 2015) was a joint venture by Tilburg University and St. Elisabeth Ziekenhuis (EZ). Its aim was to improve care at the EZ by making it more "menslievend" (loving) (Van Heijst, 2011). This aim was realized by stimulating a transformation in professional care, operational management, quality management, and policy development by anchoring, or rather re-anchoring care in the relationships between patients and their relatives on the one hand and care-providers on the other. Improvement of professional care is also a key objective of the MS Centrum Midden Brabant that was created in 2013 by physicians of the St Elisabeth and Tweesteden hospital. One of the proven instruments for the transformation of professional care is the opening up of practices of care by qualitative studies that describe their meaning (Patton, 2005), it was one of the means to stimulate transformation of care in the Professional Loving Care program. This dissertation is such a qualitative study and with that objective – the improvement and transformation of care in MS – it was integrated in the MLZ program.

This study focusses on professional care for people recently diagnosed with MS and addresses only in a remote way the other three lines of the MLZ program (i.e. the transformation of the hospital organization, the conceptualization of quality and of policy). Professional care for people with suspicion of MS is hallmarked by a series of diagnostic tests and subsequent decision-making about treatment with disease modifying therapies (DMT's). The two processes have in common that they both heavily involve the interpretation of complex statistical and biomedical information and the deliberation of risks and benefits of medical treatment. The current revised criteria for testing for MS (Polman et al., 2011) focus on the pathologies in the central nervous system (spinal cord and brain) and distinguish between "clinically isolated syndrome" and "definitive MS". Out of the three types of definitive MS, relapsing remitting MS is the most common one. This type of MS causes varied and unpredictable symptoms and sometimes may evolve after a couple of years into secondary progressive MS. In this study "MS" refers specifically to definitive relapsing remitting MS. There currently exists no cure for MS. Medical treatment may slow down the severity of relapses and the progression of the disease course. Early treatment is often recommended (Costello, Halper, Kalb, Skutnik, & Rapp, 2016). However, the efficacy of medical treatment (oral, infused, injectable) remains limited and may cause severe mild or severe adverse effects like injection site reactions, flu-like symptoms, depression, liver, thyroid, hematological abnormalities and increased risk for severe viral infections (Michel, Larochelle, & Prat, 2015). The complexity of diagnostic tests and decision-making about treatment and the life changing perspective of having this non-curable, possibly very debilitating disease make providing professional care to people that are suspected to have MS a challenging endeavor for professional and patient alike (Krahn, 2014).

The paradigm that guided the MLZ program consisted of a conceptual blend of concepts united under the term "professional loving care" (Van Heijst, 2011) and of insights from "presence theory" (A. J. Baart, 2007). The broader intellectual context of the MLZ program is a current increase of attention among Dutch and Flemish (nursing) ethicists, including Van Heijst, Vosman, & Baart (2009), Grypdonck (1997), Gastmans (2006) and others, to ethics of care. This increased attention was instigated by the book "Moral Boundaries" (1993) of Tronto that sparked interest in care as a relational and political practice that is responsive to the patients' needs and perspectives (Heier, Kohlen, & Olthuis, 2014). The integration of empirical research into ethics of care is often motivated by the responsiveness to perspectives and needs that are held in high esteem in ethics of care. Insights from empirical (qualitative) research can help health care professionals and informal care givers to understand what it means for patients to have to go through the experience of living with disease and to see how these experiences are rooted in patients' daily lives (Casterlé et al., 2011). Klaver, Elst, & Baart (2013) have summarized the critical insights of the ethics of care that were developed in the Low Countries in four points: (1) relationship-based programming, (2) recognition of situatedness and contextuality, (3) care ethics as a political–ethical discipline, and (4) theory that is empirically grounded. The first three criteria are in agreement with the international development of the ethics of care. The fourth insight is more geographically bound to the above-mentioned group of Dutch and Flemish (nursing) ethicists, although also European (health) care ethicists, including Nortvedt (2014), Kohlen (2011), and more, have also started to integrate empirical qualitative research into ethics of care.

Phenomenology and the improvement of professional care

The theoretical framework of our study is phenomenology. Phenomenology is a reflective attitude that aims at a step by step exploration of the structure and features of human experience (Moran, 2002). The basic idea of the founding father of phenomenology, Husserl, was that lived experience could be studied as an object in its own right by bracketing the everyday world, such as it is taken for granted in our natural everyday experience of it. First we present a concise picture of how phenomenology in the past and in the present has influenced and fueled reflection about good medical care. Then in the remainder of the introduction we reflect on how phenomenology and ethics of care can be merged into a phenomenological ethic of care. Halfway through the development of our thoughts on the relation between phenomenology and ethic of care, we pause, to present a review of previous literature about good care in MS and to state our research question.

The first historic movement of using phenomenology as a way to understand and improve care was anthropological medicine, a phenomenological school that flourished in the first half of the twentieth century in Germany and the Netherlands. Current conceptions of health care often operationalize good care as the product of corporate performance measured by the achievement of pre-set standards like levels of patient satisfaction. Anthropological medicine understood medical care as a delicate combination of human art and natural science, without playing the two off against each other (care as corporate business was at the time not yet on the horizon). Anthropological medicine favored a normative conception of medical care. This conception had three basic tenets (Ten Have, 1995). First it maintained foremost a holistic idea of the human person and the human body. It refused to accept materialistic and psychologist reductions as exclusive and prerogative conceptions of the human person (Dekkers, 1995). Second, this refusal opened the door to the consideration of a wide range of issues as relevant for care, including the lived body, subjectivity (Toombs, 1988), relatedness (Ten Have & Gordijn, 2014), and the very meaning of human existence itself (Martinsen & Solbakk, 2012). Finally, anthropological medicine addressed disease not only as an ensemble of causal mechanisms, but also as a way of being human and as a problem of sense-making.

Powerful current reiterations of the basic insights of anthropological medicine (including its critical stance towards reductionisms and dualisms) can be found in Carel (2013), Holmes, Murray, Perron, & Rail (2006) and Martinsen (2011). Just as a matter of background information on the topicality of this approach: in the countries surrounding the Netherlands at present we find very active groups of scholars at the intersection of medicine and phenomenology, e.g. the German physician and philosopher Fuchs (2000) and other pupils of phenomenologist Hermann Schmitz (Schmitz, Müllan, & Slaby, 2011) who are active as physicians and therapists. In Belgium we see a similar interest at Louvain's Husserl-Archives: Centre for Phenomenology and Continental Philosophy, guided by Nicholas de Warren. In both groups there is a particular interest in phenomenology, neurology and the neurosciences at large. Phenomenology transforms professional care not by the production and dissemination of technically applicable knowledge (like in the natural sciences). Rather, it aims at the development of the "habits of mind" of patients (Carel, 2012), health professionals (Greenfield & Jensen, 2010) and of researchers in health sciences (Murray, 2012) by promoting the reflective or theoretical attitude (*epochè*). This attitude enables patients, professionals and health care researchers to apprehend illness, the human person and the body as the makeup of the lived world of the patient (Finlay, 2003) instead of as biomedical objects alone.

Phenomenology and ethics of care

We stated above briefly the four critical insights of the ethics of care that forms the background of this study: (1) relationship-based programming, (2) recognition of situatedness and contextuality, (3) care ethics is a political–ethical discipline, and (4) the theory is empirically grounded. We now turn to the question how these insights can be related to phenomenology. A short answer to this question is that ethic of care and phenomenology can merge with each other when ethicists of care study relationships (first insight), situatedness (second insight) and political aspects (third insight) as *lived phenomena*. But a longer answer requires a more extensive account of the relationship between phenomenology and ethic of care. Encouragement towards a – in our eyes – sound direction for such an account can be found in works by Murray (2007, 2009, 2012, 2013, 2014) and Holmes (2004, 2006, 2015). Murray and Holmes understand phenomenological ethics as a discipline that investigates "the critical and necessary conditions that will allow for a subject to appear as an ethical being, and as the bearer of an ethical claim, whether that claim is expressed in the body or whether it is vocalized." (Murray & Holmes, 2014).

We use the work of Murray and Holmes and especially Murray's (2012) reading of Husserl (1965) to develop the four critical insights of ethics of care synopsized by Klaver, Elst, & Baart (2013) as elements of a phenomenological ethic of care. We consider, in this study, the fourth insight (the theory is empirically grounded) as dealing with the more technical aspects of such ethics (*how* to perform this kind of phenomenology). The other three insights we consider, in this study, to be more 'substantial', because they refer to the aspect of *what* can be investigated in a phenomenological ethic of care. We first turn to the more 'substantial' aspects and reflect on how relationship-based programming, recognition of situatedness and political aspects can be understood as elements of a phenomenological ethic of care. Klaver et al. (2013) rightly outlined good care as "a *stage* (our emphasis) on which the other can appear in a broader sense instead of through the lens of diagnosis or pre-set categories." The description of care as a "stage" fits well into any phenomenological framework since phenomenology aims at an description of how objects appear to people. But a more refined phenomenological understanding of care and want is needed to be able to acquire a phenomenological understanding of relationship-based programming, recognition of situatedness and political aspects. A rereading with Murray (2012) of Husserl's "Vienna lecture" of 10 may 1935 (Husserl, 1965) helped us achieve such an understanding.

The main concepts of Husserl's "Vienna lecture" are "Geist" (spirit) and "Leben" (life). The concepts of spirit and life are at the beginning of the lecture defined as the core themes of the human sciences (Geisteswissenschaften). Life and spirit refer not only to personal life but apply equally to how people live together in a community that constitutes the horizon of human experience. For Husserl life and spirit had normative connotations. At the time of the delivery of the lecture he saw the life and spirit of Europe (taken here as a specific arrangement of living together as humans) withering because of something that he called a misguided rationalism. According to Husserl this rationalism was characterized by a naïve adoption of objective knowledge of the spatiotemporal world as the sole source of knowledge (naturalism). The root of this false idea related Husserl to blindness for subjectivity as the foundation and condition for this knowledge (objectivism).

If we see phenomenology as a way of doing an ethic of care, care can be understood as a distinct way of how human living in a community is structured. We might say then that care – as a structure for living together as human persons (relationship-based programming) – meets its own spirit as a genuine human endeavor when it becomes a "stage" (Klaver et al., 2013) where the other appears as an ethical being and where consequently the conditions that enable such an appearance are in place (Murray & Holmes, 2014). The other three critical insights of ethics of care can be also approached as genuine elements of a phenomenological framework. Recognition of situatedness and contextuality (second insight) make sense as the exploration of the meaning that lived experiences gain from the lifeworld of which they are elements. But recognition may also mean the acknowledgement of the proper spirit of specific arrangements (care, often also in the form of social structures, like families and hospitals) that structure how people live together. Ethics of care as a political–ethical discipline (third insight) can be connected with Husserl's ideas about the *health condition* of human communities and of relationships. In the Vienna lecture Husserl quite bluntly stated that Europe (understood as a spiritual and living entity) is sick. Husserl was first and foremost concerned with the cultural and intellectual origins of this 'disease' (distorted rationalism affected by naturalism and objectivism). In our time also ethics of care occupies a critical stance towards society. But its concern is rather care – within our framework defined as a genuine and authentic arrangement for care receivers and providers to live and work together in a community where people can appear to each other as real persons. Kittay (2011), Tronto (1993) and other ethicists of care believe that society can be 'healed', not by reappraisal of the 'European' tradition of orderly thinking, but by liberating care from its – politically arranged – invisibility in the private corners and at the margins of society.

Literature review

Before we continue our line of thought with a reflection on the more technical aspects of a phenomenological ethic of care, we make a brief detour away from methodology and turn to the extant ethical literature on the improvement of professional care in MS and consequently to our research question. The primary initiator of research in normative accounts of MS care is without a doubt Toombs. In the 1970s – being a young woman – she was diagnosed with MS (Toombs, 1995). As a patient and as a trained philosopher she became interested in phenomenology because of her own experience as a person living with MS and her difficulty in communicating with her physicians about her illness (Toombs, 2001). Toombs sees phenomenology as a way to assure that *both* "voices" in the clinical dialogue – the biomedical voice and the voice of experience that communicates suffering – are heard (Toombs, 1988). To achieve this the philosopher from Texas launched the notion of the lived body (as shaped by Sartre, Merleau-Ponty and Zaner) as the primary paradigm for clarification of the voice of the patient. Toombs describes illness within the paradigm of the lived body as a *disruption* of the unity between self, body and world that is closely aligned with the experience of the patient of illness as existential challenge for which they seek help (Toombs, 1988). Toombs interlaces the theoretical reflections in her work with vivid short stories about her own experiences of daily living with MS, covering (non) adherence to medical treatment, moving through public space in a wheelchair, the physician–patient relationship (Toombs, 2004), travelling by plane (Toombs, 1995) and more.

Besides Toombs several other researchers have likewise explored normative perspectives on professional care in MS. In the eighties of the previous century within professional ethics for physicians it was discussed whether or not the truth should be told to patients about their MS diagnosis (Elian 1985). Finlay (2003) handles – in contrast to Toombs – experiences of daily living with MS not as anecdotes that accompany the presentation of a theoretical treatise. But rather, she prioritizes the empirical data – an interview with a young physiotherapist recently diagnosed with MS – by presenting her study as an analysis of the *lifeworld* of the participant. The meaning that MS gains from this lifeworld analysis is "disruption". Hence the empirical design of Finlay (2003) produces the same result as the more theoretical approach of Toombs. Springer (2011) investigates the relationship between the MS nurse and the patient within a framework of a Foucauldian analysis of current discourses of DMT in MS. Within this analysis, the moral commitment of the MS nurse to help the patient and to remain in relationship appears as affected by a subtle but apparent reorganization of the nursing profession by the pharmaceutical industry. This reorganization allegedly compromises the professional autonomy of the nurse, dims the supposedly weak consensus about the impact of therapies and instrumentalizes the patient-nurse relationship for commercial ends. Stahl (2013), like Toombs a researcher living with MS, situates medical images – particularly computerized axial tomography (CT) and magnetic resonance imaging (MRI) – in a political, social and economic context and outlines how the physician that is aware of the power of these images can help the patient to resignify his or her disease by putting the varied ways of embodied living with MS that the professional sees in the clinic at the disposal of the patient. Finally, Krahn (2013) argues that the construction of ethics of MS care as the application of rules about rights and duties is too narrow to cover the complex and uncertain journey that the establishment of a MS diagnosis entails for both patient and doctor. Instead, Krahn (2013) proposes care ethics as a framework for professional care in MS. He emphasizes how MS diagnosis is rather than an event, a process that is intimately tied to the lifeworld of the patient. Information about MS and treatment should be slowly integrated into this lifeworld.

Research questions

We now proceed by situating the study and by stating our research questions. Following from our phenomenological approach – an approach that sharply differentiates between an empirical and a phenomenal world – our first definition of "MS" as definitive relapsing remitting MS – a genuinely biomedical concept – needs to be complemented by a second definition that describes MS as a phenomenon in lived experience. But definitive relapsing remitting MS is a biomedical concept, so direct investigation of definitive relapsing remitting MS as a phenomenon is impossible. However, we can explore how people that received relapsing remitting MS diagnosis experience their lives. The second definition of MS that we employ in this study thus describes MS as the lived experience of people that have received the definitive relapsing remitting MS diagnosis.

Secondly, the literature discussed above shows that since the seventies (when, for example, Toombs was diagnosed with MS) within the clinical dialogue the already powerful "voice of medicine" has only become louder at the expense of the "voice of experience" (Toombs, 1988). Huge technical and medical advances – including the introduction of MRI and CT imaging technologies and the advent of DMT – in MS care have strengthened the position of the creators and owners of specialist technical and scientific knowledge (Stahl 2013). Without a doubt the rise of bioethics as the leading framework for the conceptualization of ethical care can be understood as a sincere effort to give to the operators of advanced biomedical technologies a moral context for their work. However, the emphasis of this framework on abstract principles and on active human agency as something individual obscures how physicians and patients actually live with each other and with illness in the real world (Krahn, 2014).

In this study we want to retrieve the voice of experience of living with MS by 'diving' as deep as possible into the lived experiences of people with MS. To achieve this we must embark on the performance of reduction by bracketing assumptions about many things. We mention here the three most basic ones (Toombs 1988). We need to abstain from understanding illness as a medically and socially anchored concept and to try focus instead on the ripples that mark the entry and unfolding of the body in lived experience. We need to withdraw from standardized measures of space and to investigate how places and distances get meaning by the ability to traverse them. We must also leave our ideas behind about time as displayed by the running of the clock and focus instead on bodily rhythms (fluctuations, pulsations, episodes and periodicities) and on appearances of time as spoiled, precious, feared, empty or lost. Next we will introduce Interpretative Phenomenological Analysis (IPA) as the way we use phenomenology in our qualitative empirical research. When using IPA we will follow these three understandings when applicable. The performance of reduction as the abandoning of pre-set ideas should result in the acquisition of the attitude (*epochè*) that should enable us to get an idea of what the "voice of experience" of people with MS sounds like.

Research methodology (Interpretative Phenomenological Analysis)

We now return to our discussion on the methodology of this study and continue with the more technical aspects of this methodology. *How* can a phenomenological ethics of care be performed? By dealing with this question we address the problem how such ethics are empirically grounded (fourth critical insight). In phenomenology the idea of research as the construction of a theory that explains an empirical phenomenon – the classic case is grounded theory methodology – does not apply. Rather phenomenology investigates phenomena such as they appear to persons. Phenomenology hence doesn't create theories that explain that produces insights in the basic tenets of phenomena such as they can be understood while contemplating the stirs and upheavals of lived experience. To specify: the phenomenological approach is about the lived experience as a phenomenon that to a certain extent reveals itself to perception. The research question of this study addresses the often hidden lived experiences of people with MS. Above we have broadly outlined phenomenology as a moral approach to care. But phenomenology has also manifested itself in recent decades in a variety of methods for qualitative research. One of these manifestations – IPA (Pietkiewicz & Smith, 2014; Smith, Flowers, & Larkin, 2009) – is our preferred guide for the drafting of the design of our study. We use it in an adapted form developed by Murray & Holmes (2014).

IPA was introduced in the 1990s as a new method in health psychology that could overcome the divide that existed at the time between "cognition" and "discourse analysis" (Smith, 1996). Currently IPA is also a method for research also in other fields besides psychology (Pietkiewics & Smith, 2014) including fields that approach care as a moral endeavor (Murray & Holmes, 2013, 2014). We'll give some of its characteristics: (1) The most common method in IPA for eliciting the lived experience is dialogue between participant and researcher as developed in one-on-one, semi-structured and in-depth interviews. (2) Small sample sizes (6 up to 15 participants) are thus considered appropriate for doctoral research in IPA since such sizes allow for the – quite laborious – in depth examination of similarities and differences between single cases (Pietkiewicz & Smith, 2014). Beyond these two general characteristics IPA is often defined by its three theoretical underpinnings. The first two underpinnings are phenomenology and hermeneutics. In IPA hermeneutics and phenomenology are juxtaposed as methods for phenomenological analysis. Besides *apprehension* of the interpretations of participants (Bevan 2014), hermeneutics in IPA – as a follow up step - also entails *interpretation by the researcher* as a method for the exploration of lived experience, closely related to, but also distinct from, reduction. This is the concept of the double hermeneutic. The third theoretical underpinning refers to the emphasis on the description of the idiosyncratic aspects of phenomena in the lifeworlds of individuals rather than the identification of invariant structural elements in lifeworlds of both of individuals and populations.

We have adapted IPA to our research purposes by (1) by reducing the role of the second underpinning in analysis (hermeneutics) almost to zero and (2) by adopting the linguistic-phenomenological approach of Murray (2012), Murray & Holmes (2013, 2014) to shape the first underpinning (phenomenology). In this approach, spoken language is not a tool or a means to an end, an idea that is silently implied in many IPA studies, rather language is a phenomenon that unfolds in a relational scene of address (Merleau-Ponty, 1962). Far from just data collection, the setting of the research interview is viewed in this version of IPA as an "intersubjective correlate or metaphor for the event that was originally experienced as individual" (Murray & Holmes, 2014). We adopted this version of phenomenology (including the minimalization of the role of hermeneutics) for two reasons. First, during the analysis, it appeared that the interviews didn't contain much interpretation, which hampered the application of the double hermeneutic. Second, during analysis it also gradually became clear that we were in need of a more *phenomenological* theory about the linguistic nature of our data than existing IPA theory and studies could provide. With the approach of Murray (2012), Murray & Holmes (2013, 2014) we were able to address this need. The third underpinning of IPA, ideography, we left unchanged.

In the fourth year of the MLZ program (2012) five MLZ associates created a four member analysis team and a three member interview team to explore the lived experiences of people with a recent (< 2 years) definitive relapsing remitting MS diagnosis. Two MLZ associates where included in both teams. The analysis team prepared for the interviews and analysis cycle by drafting an interview guide that addressed diagnosis, work, private life, and medical care. In this way we wanted to explore illness and care as phenomena in the varied social structures that make up the lifeworld of people with MS. Ten patients recruited from the database of the MS Centrum Midden Brabant gave consent to participate in one on one interviews in their homes. Each participant was interviewed once. The interviews lasted at least one hour up to more than two hours and were recorded with an audio recorder. The recordings were transcribed by two members of the interview team and secretaries of the MS Centrum Midden Brabant and entered in the software package ATLAS.ti version 6.1 for further analysis. In table 1 we present the profile of the participants.

Table 1: Profile of the participants

Participant	Interviewer	Gender	Age
#06 'Kathy'	Archie de Ceuninck	F	27
#03 'Lucilia'	Daphne Frijlink	F	30
#09 'Shayne'	Archie de Ceuninck**	F	31
#01 'Livia'	Archie de Ceuninck	F	33
#05 'Lawrence'*	Archie de Ceuninck	M	35
#10 'Renata'	Archie de Ceuninck	F	41
#08 'Savina'	Frans J. H. Vosman**	F	43

#07 'Andrea'	Frans J. H. Vosman	F	45
#02 'Ricky'*	Daphne Frijlink	M	46
#04 'Katherine'*	Daphne Frijlink	F	51

* Partner present at the interview at the request of the participant

** Member of the analysis team *and* the interview team.

Outline

This study is outlined according to the second critical insight of the ethic of care that situatedness and contextuality need to be recognized (Klaver et al., 2013). In four consecutive chapters, three lived social frameworks (Husserl, 1965) are explored. Given the fact that the onset of MS occurs commonly in the most productive years of the patients (Hunter, 2016) we included in this study besides professional care in MS also family and occupation as two other significant topics, i.e. two additional social networks wherein people with MS experience illness and care. In chapter 1 (the process of diagnosis) and chapter 2 (decision making on and use of disease modifying therapies (DMTs) we focus on professional care in MS. In chapter 3 the situatedness of MS as a family issue comes into view. In chapter 4 we zoom in on the problem of MS and paid work. We will present the goal of each chapter under the label of the exploration of the patient perspective in the specific situation that is addressed in the respective chapter. With this label we denote the phenomenological analyses of the lived experience of illness and care in the mode of research that we have outlined above. The sequence of the chapters is interlaced with four excursuses that present each a longer fragment from the audio transcriptions that is meant to magnify the main insights from the preceding chapter. In the section that follows the fourth excursus, these insights are incorporated into a discussion that concludes this study.

.

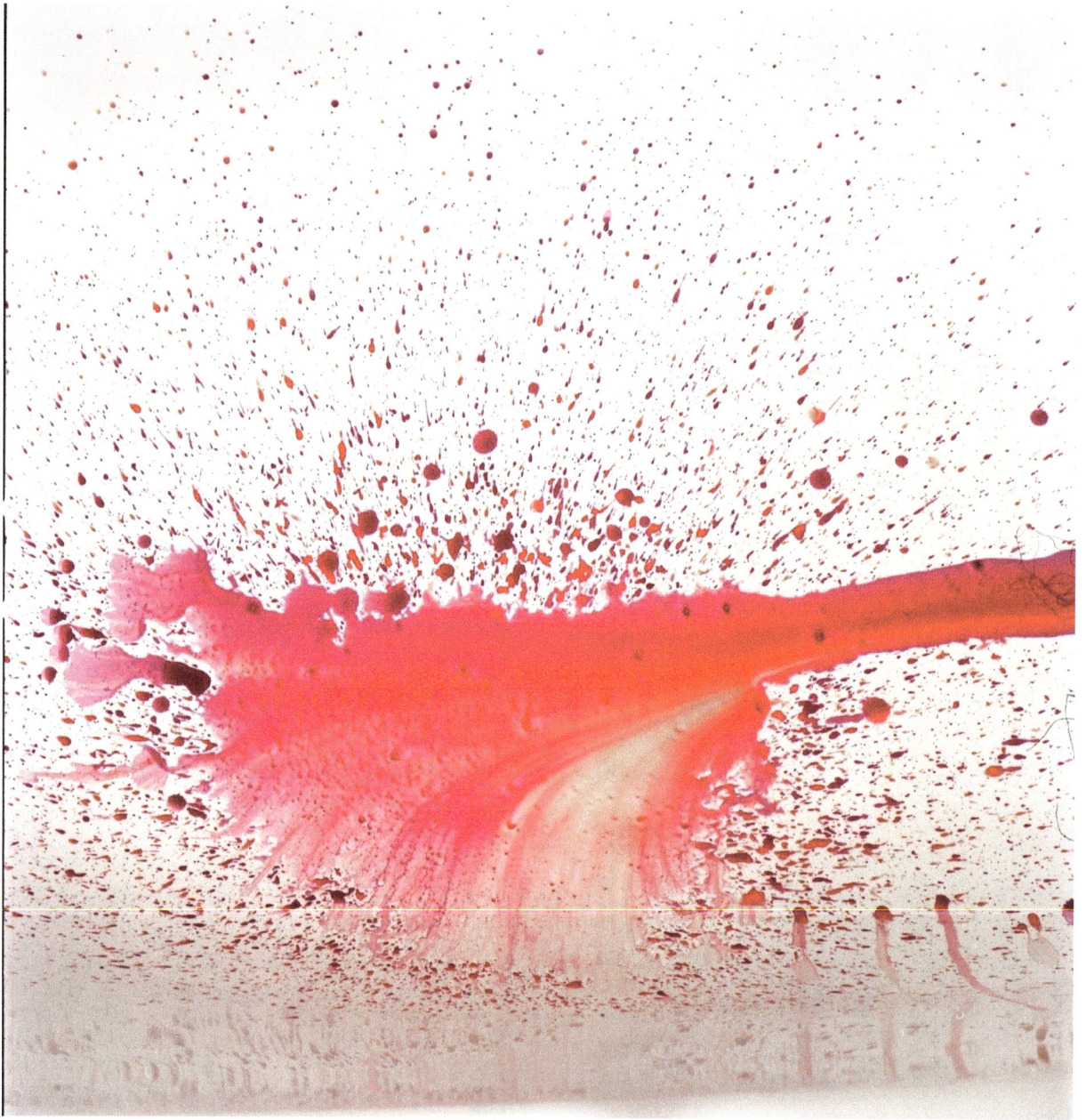

1. THE PROCESS OF DIAGNOSIS

Rationale, aims and objectives: The recent history of practices of disclosure of MS diagnoses reflects the transition from paternalistic to patient-centred care (PCC). Numerous concepts have been developed to implement this model of medicine in clinical practice. In PCC, the importance of the patient perspective is paramount. This paper offers a phenomenological examination of the patient perspective on testing for MS. Methods: Ten people diagnosed with MS were interviewed in open, in depth interviews. Transcriptions were analyzed using a phenomenological approach. Results: One main theme "Varying perceptions of the diagnosis" and four subthemes were identified. The subthemes are: (a) increased awareness of the body, (b) alienating spaces, (c) intensified perceptions of time and, (d) intensified perceptions of medical personnel. Conclusions: The analysis of the patient perspective on the process of MS diagnosis shows intensified and wavering perceptions of body, place, time and medical employees. Accepting patient perceptions as constitutive elements of the doctor-patient relationship may help clinicians make care for persons that are being tested for MS more patient-centred. As a concrete proposal for improvement of current practices we suggest avoiding the transmission of the test results at the first meeting of patient and doctor. Doctor and patient should get acquainted with each other and each other's perspectives at the beginning of the diagnostic trajectory and together journey towards its conclusion.

Ceuninck van Capelle, A. de, Visser, L. H., & Vosman, F. J. H. (2016): Developing Patient-Centred Care for Multiple Sclerosis (MS). Learning from Patient Perspectives on the process of MS diagnosis. European Journal for Person Centered Healthcare 4 (4) doi: 10.5750/ejpch.v4i4.1191.

Introduction

The past decades have seen a major transition in the field of reflection on the physician-patient relationship during the process of MS diagnosis (Raphael, Hawkes, & Bernat, 2013). This transition first began in the 1960s (Morgan & Yoder, 2012). In the eighties scholars (Elian & Dean, 1985; Sencer, 1988) as well as patients (Burnfield, 1984; Toombs, 1988) started to question the paternalist approach to MS in which physicians decided on their own discretion whether or not to reveal a MS diagnosis. An unpublished survey amongst doctors, quoted in a brief report (Levine, 1983), revealed that most doctors that delayed diagnosis disclosure had wanted to reveal the diagnosis in due time. Reasons that hampered them in doing so included the unpredictable and fluctuant disease course, concerns about the patients' capacity to understand the nature of the illness and, finally, the patients' ability to cope with the illness emotionally. Against these justifications, critics of the paternalistic model highlighted the right of patients to know their own health condition and to reflect personally about options for treatment. Within only a couple of years, the paternalist model of medicine was replaced by other models, amongst them PCC. In PCC the physician provides the patient with adequate medical information and encourages his or her autonomy (Morgan & Yoder, 2012; Raphael et al., 2013).

The changed relationship between providers and recipients of care in PCC has produced several specific and detailed models of this relationship. We mention here three frequently employed models. One leading model of the patient-doctor relation is shaped by the concept of the market (McLaughlin, 2009). In (the metaphor of) the market, the patient is a consumer that makes choices guided by personal preferences, values and needs. The doctor is first and foremost a *supplier* of medical care. Another model of the patient-doctor relationship is shaped by the concept of active citizenship (Newman & Tonkens, 2011). Official policies aimed at the reduction of demand for public health care promote this model. This reduction is expected to be achieved by encouraging the patient to maintain a healthy and active lifestyle. In this patient–doctor relationship, the *prevention* of illness is as important as the *treatment* of illness. Finally, the concept of shared decision making (Barry & Edgman-Levitan, 2012) sees the doctor and the patient as a team that works towards the best medical outcome. This concept focuses on moments of medical decision making, where different choices may lead to different and irreversible results.

Aside from a short report by June Halper, in which she expresses her endorsement of comprehensive care such as implementation of PCC for MS, practices of MS care haven't been studied or discussed from the angle of PCC. In this article we address this gap. We do this by exploring the patient perspective on the process of MS diagnosis. We assume that PCC in MS must account for the patient perspective on this particular illness. MS care is not *only* addressed to bundles of cells, nerves, tissues and fluids. Doctors and other providers of care serve *also* fellow human beings who feel, perceive, think and hope just like anyone else. Providers of PCC for people with MS should therefore embrace how persons with MS perceive their condition, no matter what specific model of the doctor-patient relationship – consumerism, active citizenship, shared decision-making or another PCC model – actually guides their practices.

The patient perspective is not born in a vacuum. We assume that what the patient perceives, feels, thinks and hopes is for a considerable part determined by what the patient is *allowed* to perceive, feel, think and hope. In other words we always assume a political context that moulds personal experience (Fisher, 2007). The patient perspective in clinical doctor-patient encounters is not a natural phenomenon. Cultural and political concepts of body, care , patient and the objectives of professional intervention may hinder rather than promote the inclusion of the patient perspective in practices of care (Greenfield & Jensen, 2010; Krahn, 2014). Therefore we believe that doctors need to recognize, promote and protect the patient perspective *actively* (Martinsen, 2011). In a similar manner researchers of the patient perspective should also be sensitive to the conditions that stimulate or subdue patient expression of perception, feelings, thoughts and hopes.

Methods

Our study began in 2012. We used purposeful sampling to include people with a definitive relapsing remitting MS diagnosis who had received their diagnosis a maximum of two years previously. Recruitment was carried out by approaching patients from the records of a hospital's ambulatory MS care unit until we reached 10 participants (De Ceuninck van Capelle et al., 2015). This number was in line with our aim of carrying out an explorative study and congruent with the demands of the particular phenomenological method that we had adopted; *Interpretative Phenomenological Analysis* (IPA) (Murray & Holmes, 2014; Smith et al., 2009).

In 2013 three interviewers, the first and third author and a resident neurologist, conducted conversational interviews at the homes of the participants. The interviews were conducted in Dutch, the native language of the participants and of the interviewers and researchers. Following an open, explorative approach, we encouraged the participants to talk about what mattered most to them (Hodge, 2008). The interviewers made use of a concise topic list that included work, personal situation, diagnosis and care. The participants were encouraged to prioritize, add or discard topics on their own accord. The ethical committee of the St. Elisabeth Hospital in Tilburg approved the research and the patients gave informed consent for participation.

Data was gathered from 13 people: 10 people with MS and three partners that were asked by the person with MS to assist them with the interview. We granted these requests, as is common in qualitative research on illness (Sakellariou, Boniface, & Brown, 2013). All participants resided in the Netherlands and the patients and participating partners were Caucasian. The people with MS were aged 27-51 years. Table 1 shows the profiles of the participants.

Table 1: Profile of the participants

Participant #	Pseudonym	Interviewer	Gender	Age
6	Kathy	1st author	F	27
3	Lucilia	DF	F	30
9	Shayne	1st author	F	31
1	Livia	1st author	F	33
5	Lawrence	1st author	M	35
10	Renata	1st author	F	41
8	Savina	2nd author	F	43
7	Andrea	2nd author	F	45
2	Ricky	DF	M	46
4	Katherine	DF	F	51

The analysis was guided by the phenomenological, hermeneutical and ideographic underpinnings of IPA (Smith et al., 2009). Data analysis consisted of three stages of inductive analysis of the digital audio files. In the first stage, shortly after each interview, the authors and a postdoc researcher added, independently from each other, preparatory notes in Dutch in the right margins of the transcripts. Within these notes, each researcher recorded free associations, pieces of theory, questions and possible related topics against specific excerpts of the transcript. Subsequently the transcripts and notes were discussed in six plenary meetings. The cycle of interviewing, noting and discussing was repeated after each interview until the entire sample of 10 interviews was completed. In early 2013, a general meeting of the three authors at which emergent threads were identified concluded the first stage. In 2013 and 2014 the first author entered the second stage by reworking the results of the first stage into a network of in vivo coded codes, supported by data analysis software Atlas.ti version 6.2, using a constant comparison method. The third stage started in the autumn of 2014, guided by the network of codes and the methodological underpinnings of IPA the first author identified one main theme and four subthemes on the experienced diagnostic process.

Results

One main theme and four subthemes were identified by the analysis. The main theme is: Varying perceptions of the diagnosis. The subthemes are: (a) increased awareness of the body, (b) alienating spaces, (c) intensified perceptions of time and, (d) intensified perceptions of medical personnel. Below the main theme and its four subthemes are described accompanied by illustrative quotes.

Varying perceptions of the diagnosis

The trajectories that led to the definitive diagnosis varied. Some participants (Shayne, Livia, Lawrence, Renata and Andrea) received their definitive diagnosis just a few days after the occurrence of the complaints that had started the chain of medical tests that would lead to the diagnosis. For others (Savina and Katherine), the disclosure of the definitive diagnosis was preceded by two years of complaints for which no physician had found a conclusive diagnosis. And for a third group, (Kathy, Lucilia and Ricky), the definitive diagnosis was preceded by a period of several months that followed the delivery of a provisional diagnosis.

The experience of feeling shocked after receiving the diagnosis (either provisional or definitive) was common:

"And then the doctor said [while showing the images of the MRI scan]: 'This is not good'. And when he said the word 'MS', I went off the grid, I was no longer present, so to say. So my aunt took over from me and started to ask all kinds of questions. I could only think of wheelchairs and expected to die within the year." {6:7} Kathy

In combination with the feeling of shock, two other perceptions of the diagnosis appeared as well. Some participants (Kathy, Lucilia and Renata) tried to distance themselves from their illness by hoping for a mild course:

"Eight months before [I received my definitive diagnosis] I had already had one lesion. But we decided to look at it from the bright side: 'It is just one lesion. Period.' They said to us: 'You could have MS, but we'll know for sure only after the incidence of more lesions.' Anyway, we didn't search for information about MS. We didn't want to deal with that. We thought to ourselves: 'If we're going to search for information it [MS], it comes far too close.'" {3:7} Lucilia

For Katherine and Savina the diagnosis invoked a sense of relief and meant the conclusion of a long period of confusion and tiresome medical examinations:

Two years ago, things suddenly came together. (…) And that brought me a sense of peace. Well, peace might not be the proper word, that brought me clarity, yes, peace indeed. Before the diagnosis I thought: 'I'm so tired because of 'this or that' …' But now the diagnosis [as the explanation for how I often feel] is known." Savina {8:143}

For Kathy, Lucilia and Savina the diagnosis appears respectively as a complete surprise, as a threatening thought that is kept at distance and as the conclusion of a long and exhaustive journey towards a medical explanation for experienced complaints.

(a) Increased awareness of the body

For the participants that were diagnosed shortly after their first complaints, the first period following this event was a time of increased awareness of their bodies:

"You get acquainted with your body and you actually have to do so, too. Last year, I had a bladder infection. I thought: 'Well, if I have to deal with this for the rest of my life …., I don't like that at all.' But after a while you realize: 'It's just a bladder infection, it's not part of it [MS], this just happens. And almost every night, when I'm watching television in a lazy position, my legs start to tingle. Then I think: 'Let's get up, walk and move a bit', and then the tingle goes away. The same with my hands. Just move them a bit, and that nasty feeling goes away. All those kinds of tricks, you know. {1:89} Livia

After the establishment of the diagnosis, participants test its usefulness as a frame for constructing a new personal understanding of their bodily experiences. Both before and after the diagnosis the body is perceived with reservation and a degree of suspicion.

(b) Alienating spaces

All participants recounted alienating experiences of space before, during and even after the delivery of the diagnosis:

"The MRI [scanner] is a narrow space filled with noise. What I always did [when being there] was improvise a melody on the patterns in the noise. I did that very much on purpose. Because it sucks big time being in there. Very narrow there and very loud, as if you're working at a construction site. For people, that is very restricting and very frightening." {6:143} Kathy

And then the nurses came to me, while I was taking shower. I: In the shower?! P: Yes, but don't worry, they knocked on the door first. [They said]: 'Miss, in a little bit the doctor will arrive with the results of the tests. You have to call your family.' Well, I felt like the ground was moving, because I thought that they had found a brain tumour. (…) After a while the neurologist came and said to us: "Yes, come with me to my office." (…) I had literally been banging my head against the wall [of the shower]: 'My daughter is 1,5 years old. If I have a brain tumour, who's going to take care of her?'"? {9:37} Shayne

[After my dismissal from the hospital] I stayed at home for a week. After that I went back to the office to work in the mornings. I really wanted that, because I was going mad being here at home. I had a nice, new house but I wasn't able to enjoy it at all. So I thought: 'If I only had something to do ….' {1:29} Livia

Before and after the diagnosis participants become unsettled and move through hospital spaces in which they feel out of control. The patient wants to belong somewhere and feel solid ground again.

(c) Intensified perceptions of time

Some participants mentioned slowing down (Livia) as well as acceleration (Andrea) of time:

> On Wednesday morning I got a brain MRI. And when I returned from that, a nurse approached me and said to me: 'The neurologists wants a family consultation. I can't give any details.' Well, at that moment my world ceased to exist. It was a hard blow. I thought: 'They have identified a tumor.' It took 2,5 hours before the meeting started. Those 2,5 hours were like hell." {1:7} Livia

> "On Tuesday I was still cycling to work. And on Wednesday I was tied to an infusion [to receive treatment to prevent exacerbation]. So the intermediate period [between onset and diagnosis] was very, very short. It overwhelms you, your environment, everybody." {7:72} Andrea

Alongside the experiences of unsettlement run intensified perceptions of time. Astonishment and fear interrupt the ordinary pace of life.

(d) Intensified perceptions of medical personnel

Most participants retained memories of particular persons that they met or thought about during the period of diagnostic testing. For each participant these could be different persons. The illustrations of the previous subthemes showed how the walls of Livia's house made her long for the company of her colleagues and how the first thought of Shayne after the announcement of the meeting was devoted to her 1,5 years old daughter. One particular person that all participants kept memories of was the person of the physician that brought them the bad news. Their impression of the physician could be positive or negative, we will give one example of each case:

> "He showed me the screen and said: 'Don't be afraid, you don't have cancer. But those white spots show degeneration of myelin. That means that you have MS.' (...) At first, I was happy. After all, stress didn't appear to be the cause [of my complaints]. But then, I became scared. (...) Looking back, the doctor did a good job, he explained it well." {4:70} Katherine

> "The neurologist on duty delivered the bad news directly and at once. I find him a horrible man and we didn't find any common ground. We had a lot of questions but we

hardly got any answers. At the conclusion of the meeting he said: 'Miss, the glass is half full or half empty, depending on how you look at it. (…) Make the best out of it.' We were horrified, although at a fundamental level, he's right of course. But he didn't respond to any of our emotions [of grief and distress]. {7:129} Andrea

The intensified perceptions of physicians focus particularly at their voices during the explanation of the conclusions of the diagnostic tests. Either directly or after some time participants also perceive how medical personnel related to their situation at the time.

Discussion

Combined these results provide valuable insights into the patient perspective on the process of MS diagnosis. The findings corroborate with those of older studies on the lived experience of MS that depict it as a journey into the unknown (Barker-Collo, Cartwright, & Read, 2006; Koopman & Schweitzer, 1999; Miller, 1997). They confirm the significance, also identified by earlier studies, of the moment of the delivery of the diagnosis (Barker-Collo et al., 2006; Solari et al., 2007). But the findings also point at other, not previously identified aspects of the process of MS diagnosis: intensified perceptions of spaces, bodies, time course and specific others. A possible explanation for the strong focus on the disclosure of the diagnosis in previous research might be the idea that patients have the right to know the nature of their condition. The focus at disclosure of the diagnosis that comes with this concept has probably caused negligence towards the events that precede and follow disclosure. However, the findings of our study show that the 'before' and 'after' of the disclosure of the results of the diagnostic tests deeply matter from a patient perspective. Not only the result, but also the process of MS diagnosis matters.

One of the not previously identified aspects of the process of MS diagnosis is the variation in experienced space and time. This implies that although from an objective point of view it seems that providers of care and patients are at the same time and place in the same hospital, from a subjective point of view this might not be the case. Two hours in and average working day for a busy and occupied nurse or physician often pass without notice but for patients waiting for life changing results they may last for eternity. An MRI scanner is to a skilled technician a complicated but understandable instrument to do his job, but may to patients resemble a coffin and a harbinger of death. Hence, the 'gap' between the experienced time and place of medical employees and of patients might be considerable. A serious assessment of moments that offer genuine opportunities to bridge this gap might help get patients and professionals more synchronized. We think that the recommendations of Solari (Solari et al., 2007) for communicating the diagnosis and of Krahn (Krahn, 2014) for addressing the uncertainties and feelings during the process of diagnosis may well apply here. Differences in experienced space and time as well as the use of complex medical technologies may seriously burden interactions between care givers and care providers. Becoming more aware of the factors that impede communication may help patients and doctors to protect and continue their relationship with their patients just when it matters most.

Another important finding is the prominence of perceptions of particular others and notably of the physician that delivers the result of the diagnostic tests. This finding was unexpected and suggests that the collective image of the physician as the professional that controls complex medical technology needs to be complemented by the physician as a person or subject whom patients feel related to, for better or for worse. This study confirms the finding of previous studies that good information at the moment is disclosure is crucial. However, delivering MS diagnosis is not only about the message, but also about the relation between messenger and the recipient. Patients perceive strongly to what extent the person of the physician is capable of connecting with them and their worries about their lives and future, including their worries about the impact of MS in their relational networks of family, work and friends. Although a note of caution is due here: we think that attention to the relationship between physician and patient – a platform that conveys not only the communication of medical matters but also the consideration of social consequences of illness – facilitates and enhances the 'performance' of their roles of providers and receivers of care.

In the introduction we raised the point that we assume that what the patient perceives, feels, thinks and hopes is partially conditioned by social context. Indeed testing for serious neurological illnesses like MS takes place in such a context. The hospital is a place with its own rules. Once the patient is admitted to this place he or she is expected to adhere to the protocols and procedures that are supposed to facilitate the delivery of the best care possible. The understanding and application of these procedures (including testing for MS) requires intensive medical training. Although physicians may try to overcome the gap between medical experts and lay people by informing patients as good as they can, there always looms imbalance of power between providers and receivers of care. Because of lack of control or lack of knowledge, patients may feel overwhelmed and constrained to express their own concerns (Van Heijst, 2011). Mutual acknowledgement of physician and patient alike of the fact that these feelings may be part of the patient experience of being tested for MS, may enhance the acknowledgement and inclusion of the patient perspective in care for people with MS.

Notwithstanding the growing attention to the relevance of the patient perspective, directives, codes of professional conduct and laws that guide these practices display a conception of medicine that remains primarily biomedical. Our findings reflect this reality. At the center of the patient experience of MS diagnosis stands the medical approach conveyed by the physical space of the hospital and especially subjugation to magnetic resonance imaging. In the patient experience of testing for MS, the hospital and magnetic resonance imaging are viewed as profoundly personal issues. The hospital and the MRI scanner are perceived as alienating and (life) threatening spaces. Participants had (temporarily) intensified perceptions of their body, of time and of other persons, notably hospital employees. However, the participants seem to have noticed little awareness from the side of hospital employees for the meanings that being tested for MS held to them.

We surely don't want to dispute the professional duty of any medical practitioner to discern which elements in the story of patients are medically relevant and which are not. But the physician that understands the patient perspective not only as a possible source of medical information, but also as a constitutive element of the patient-doctor relationship, should embrace the medically relevant as well as the not biomedically relevant elements of this perspective. For the patient, illness is an undivided, complex and often very vague aggregate of fears about the future, grieving about a broken health, bodily sensations, negative and positive social experiences and perhaps much more. We believe that clinicians that advocate PCC in MS should embrace all these aspects. But, admitting these aspects into the physician-patient relationship requires courage and creativity from both sides.

To summarize the findings which have arisen in this study: from the patient perspective, during the process of diagnosis, the world of the patient becomes a contested place. The body feels different and doesn't move like it used to do, which hampers self-confidence and self-reliance. The places where the patient is brought to are unknown and full of potential threats. The world of the patient and that of the surrounding professionals are not always synchronized. The application of PCC in the process of MS diagnosis can be advanced if clinicians accept the whole patient perspective, medical, social and emotional, as a constituent in the doctor-relationship. Since relational medical practices don't happen in neutral spaces but rather in a socio-political space that emphasizes the biomedical model of medicine, this acceptance needs to be actively sought.

Limitations of this study This study has several limitations in terms of scope and design. The small size of the dataset means that the presented picture of the patient perspective on MS diagnosis is in need of complementation. The trajectories that participants have followed towards their diagnosis appear to be highly variable and affected by many contingent factors, including biological course, attentiveness of the environment, the selected medical interventions and tests and opinions of the patient on health and illness. To develop a more complete picture of the patient perspective on MS diagnosis, additional studies with more specific and perhaps also larger samples are necessary.

Recommendations for the medical practice of diagnosing MS The findings of this study show the patient perspective on being tested for MS and explore how this perspective can be integrated in the doctor-patient relationship that frames the management of the diagnostic process. Technical aspects, pace of the advancement of diagnostic tests and lack of control may impede patients to perceive being the process of MS diagnosis as a relational process which patient and doctor move through together. The process and the result of diagnostic tests for MS should therefore not be considered as separate entities. Preferably the meeting of the disclosure of the tests' results should not be the first time that the patient and the physician see each other. Scheduling a meeting at the beginning of the process with the physician that is likely to tell the results may be a simple but effective step towards a physician-patient relationship in which a shared view on the patient perspective – with its medical and non-medical aspects alike – is a constituent element. At the same time we believe that such a step – as simple as it is – is a significant step towards PCC in the process of MS diagnosis.

"I was glad that he allowed me to go home to fetch my belongings."[1]

"And then my general practitioner (GP) said something to me like:

'Well I prefer to send you to the hospital three times for nothing rather than one time too late.'

She immediately called the neurology department of the Tweestedenziekenhuis and they considered it appropriate for me to come by. After I had returned home [from my visit to the GP] I told my partner that I had to leave for the hospital. That was kind of a shock. I called a friend who came over instantly and she drove with me to the hospital. There they took blood samples and the assistant of the neurologist did some tests, again with those instruments [like the GP did], and then the neurologist himself arrived. He repeated the tests and indeed I had no feeling in my upper and lower legs and my feet and my reflex response was slower than normal. And he left and he came back and said:

'I have good news and bad news.'

And I said:

'Yes, and?'

He said:

'I can't tell you right away what it is.'

Because his first thought were about a hernia because with that comes an impingement and tingling and also because he had heard the story of the delivery [of my daughter]. And then he said:

'You can't stay here. I really have to send you to the Elisatbeth Ziekenhuis.'

I said:

'Why?'

'I want you this very evening to get hospitalized so that you can enter the scan first thing in the morning. Otherwise they will put you on a waiting list and this can't wait.'

Well that was a kind of setback. Well, of course I hadn't had dinner, it was already seven o'clock in the evening so I had asked him if I could go home for a moment to fetch my stuff and to eat something. And then he said:

'In that case I delay your hospitalization a bit.'

That was very sweet of him. And so that Tuesday night I was hospitalized. [P9:13-23]

The previously introduced distinction between the "biomedical voice" and "the voice of experience" (Frank, 2000; Toombs, 1988) may serve well as a point of departure for a reflection on this fragment that is meant to situate the previous chapter in the framework of our study. In Toombs (1988) the biomedical voice is described as "couched in the technical language of objective clinical data – blood counts, electrocardiogram interpretations, genetic screening results, and so forth – and details the medical history (what is occurring in terms of the effect of disease/pathology on the body)." The voice of experience recounts according to Toombs "the life disruption caused by the medical problem – what is happening in terms of its impact on this particular person and those with whom s/he is most intimately involved."

---

[1] The quote has been slightly adapted to fit the format of the titles of the excursuses.

It is not difficult to apply this distinction to the interview setting. In this setting participant #9 (Sayne) tried to produce for the interviewer a meaningful account of her hospitalization. This already is an important observation: as researchers we do not get an unmediated view on a phenomenon. A story is told in the context of a (short-term) relationship, that of the interview. This mediation does not mean that a phenomenon does not show itself, it means that it shows itself as a story, relationally adapted to the circumstantial context. The presence of the two voices *within* the account of the participant #9 is obvious. The voice of medicine is (extremely well) 'audible' in the swift referral to the hospital. This referral reflects the professional judgment of the GP and the neurology department that Shayne's physical complaints may point to an acute and serious health problem. Other characteristics of this 'voice' are the taking of blood samples, the tests, the instruments and the rendering of Shayne's body (reflexes) and biography (the event of the birth of her daughter) in objective cause-and-effect terms of disease/pathology of the body. Shayne has a twofold attitude towards the "voice of medicine" in the event of her hospitalization. On the one hand she readily accepts her hospitalization as a sincere and necessary effort to prevent het situation from possibly getting worse. She is hence prepared to comply with the request to go to the hospital swiftly and to undergo medical examination there. But on the other hand there is also a feeble indication that Shayne feels that – the also present – "voice of experience" is in danger of getting lost.

But before we reconstruct this concern, we first turn to the "voice of experience" that is also present in the fragment. "What is happening in terms of its impact on this particular person and those with whom s/he is most intimately involved" is clearly visible in the shock that affects Shayne and her partner when it becomes clear that the GP and the hospital classify Shayne's physical complaints as an emergency case. During the interview we didn't explore the substance of this shock in more detail any further. Another element of "the voice of experience" surfaces in the phrase "those instruments". That phrase expresses distance and a feeling of alienation that may emerge while being examined with instruments of which the purpose and the efficacy is hardly known. The voice of experience finally is also evident in the conclusion of the fragment when Shayne recounts how the announcement of her hospitalization betrayed her expectations. Feelings of being tired, hungry and devoid of the personal belongings that are needed to sleep well conclude "the voice of experience" in Shayne's account of her hospitalization.

Now we have outlined the "voice of experience" in the fragment we can also reconstruct the other side of Shayne's attitude towards the "voice of medicine" in the event of her hospitalization. There is a feeble indication that Shayne feels that the "voice of experience" that runs parallel with the hospitalization remains largely unnoticed. In Shayne's account, the voice of experience and the voice of medicine almost don't interfere. But at the end of the fragment the two voices 'contact' each other when the neurologist delays hospitalization to give Shayne some time for preparation. We think that Shayne qualifies this delay as "sweet" not only because her weariness and hunger at the moment of her request. With the acknowledgement of weariness and hunger there is also a kind of tacit recognition of the impact of the advice to go to the emergency care unit, the examination with strange medical instruments and the setback of the hospitalization. In the introduction we defined care as a genuine and authentic arrangement for care receivers and providers to live and work together in a community where people can appear to each other as real persons. This is exactly what we see happening at the conclusion of the fragment. The delay involved the recognition of what the course of events had meant to Shayne as a person and allowed at the same time the neurologist to appear to Shayne as a "sweet" person that not only did what was necessary from a medical point of view but also from the perspective of medicine as a human endeavor (Ten Have 1995).

The reading of a patient account of medical care in terms of the two "voices" such as we just did with Shayne's account of her hospitalization can also be applied to the patient accounts that constituted the basis of the previous chapter. In these accounts the voice of medicine and the voice of experience run parallel with each other and – in a few cases – touch upon each other. What also becomes evident is that within a framework of care defined as a relational network wherein people can appear to each other as real persons, the focus of good care is different. Good care is in this framework not measured in terms of "centeredness" on the patient but rather defined by the quality of the relational network that supplies for the critical and necessary conditions to make ethical care happen (Murray & Holmes 2014). Hence in phenomenology as a moral approach to care, the receiver and the provider of medical care are of equal importance. In the previous chapter and in Shayne's account, the receiver and the provider of care appeared as respectively the passive and the active side of medical interaction. This is how the 'roles' of patient and physician are usually are assigned (by medical professionals) in medical theory and practice. In the next chapter, however, we will see that a phenomenological exploration of a second case of professional care in MS – DMT – indicates that this way of assigning roles rules out instances in which it are patients who assume (or even capture) the *active* part.

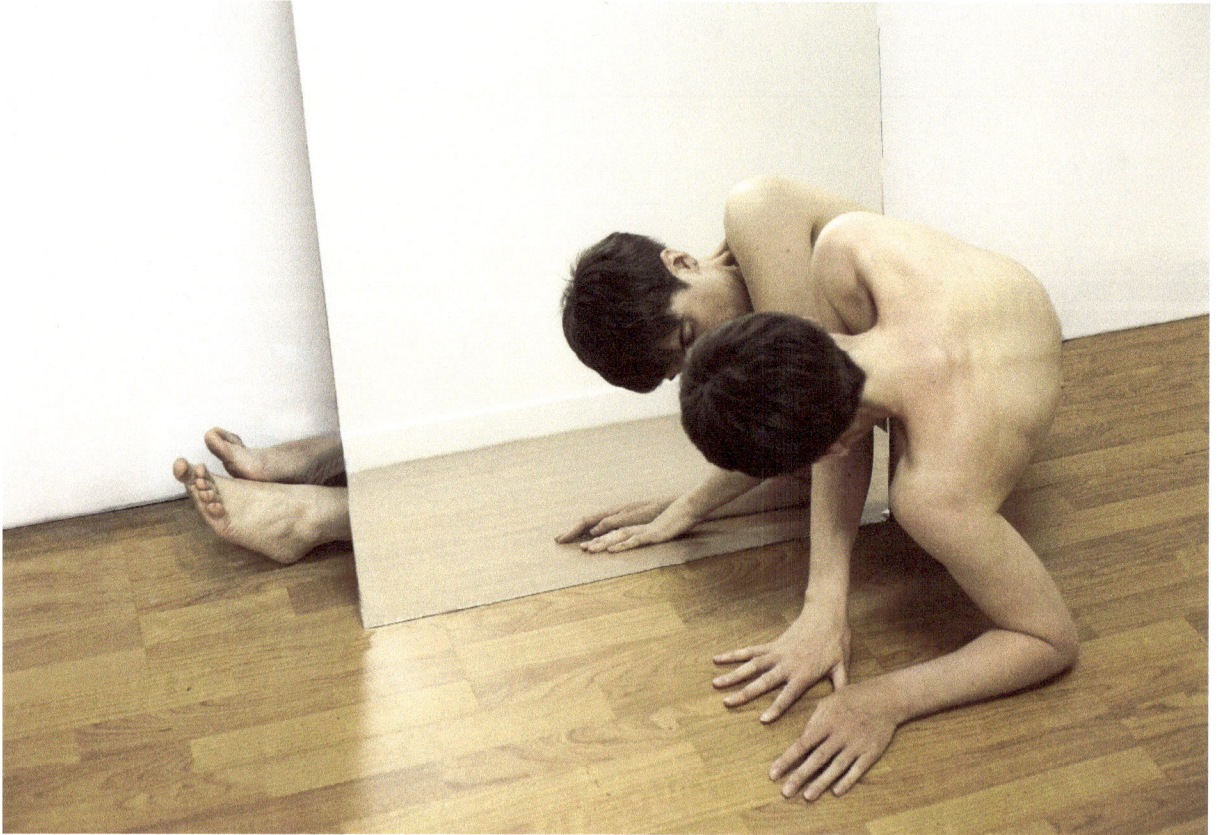

2. THE PROCESS OF DECISION-MAKING ON MODIFYING THERAPIES (DMT'S) IN MS

Background: Physicians commonly advise patients to begin disease modifying therapies (DMT's) shortly after the establishment of a Multiple Sclerosis (MS) diagnosis. Research on the patient perspective in the decision-making process on DMT's for MS is scarce. Objective: To explore the patient perspective on using DMT's for MS. Methods: Ten participants with a recent (< 2 years) relapsing remitting MS diagnosis were interviewed. Seven of them used DMT's at the time of the interview. All interviews were transcribed and analyzed using a hermeneutical-phenomenological approach. Results: Four themes emerged: (1) Constant confrontation with the disease, (2) Managing inevitable decline, (3) Hope for improvement, and, (4) Taking DMT's as a social experience. The themes show that patients associate the recommendation to begin DMT's (especially injectable DMT's) with views about their bodies as well as their hopes about the future. Both considering and adhering to treatment are experienced by patients as not only matters of individual and rational deliberation but also as activities that are lived within in a web of relationships with relatives and friends. Conclusion: From the patient perspective, the use of DMT's is not the purely rational, individual experience it is commonly conceived as being in our current understanding of the decision-making process on DMT's. More attention to DMT's as relational and lived phenomena will improve our understanding of the process of decision-making for DMT's in MS.

Ceuninck van Capelle, A. de, Meide, H. van der, Vosman, F. J. H., & Visser, L. H. (2016): A qualitative study assessing patient perspectives in the process of decision-making on disease modifying therapies (DMT's) in Multiple Sclerosis (MS). In revision at PLOS ONE.

Introduction

Multiple sclerosis (MS) is a chronic and usually progressive condition that affects the brain and spinal cord (Compston & Coles, 2008). It is typically diagnosed in young adults. Most patients experience the onset of their illness as the manifestation of fatigue, visual problems, bladder problems, distortion of sensory capacity, and electric sensations in limbs and spine on neck flexion. There is no definitive diagnostic test for MS. Five different types have been identified and in about 80% of patients the disease starts with relapsing-remitting MS (Compston & Coles,

2008). Relapsing-remitting MS is characterized by periods of episodic relapses in which a sudden onset or increase in symptoms occurs followed by a full or partial recovery. Over time, mostly around 40 years of age, 65% of the patients with MS enter the secondary progressive phase which may bring serious physical and cognitive disability (Compston & Coles, 2008) The psychological and social consequences of MS are manifold, including increased risks of depression, divorce and unemployment (Pfleger, Flachs, & Koch-Henriksen, 2010a, 2010b).

Although there is no cure for MS, several disease-modifying therapies (DMT's) have become available. Early intervention is generally recommended to limit future disease progression (Derwenskus, 2011). The most common first line DMT's for MS in the Netherlands are the ABCNR medicines: interferon beta 1a (Avonex), administered weekly, interferon beta 1b (Betaferon), administered every other day, glatiramer acetate (Copaxone), administered daily or three times a week, and interferon beta 1a (Rebif), administered three times per week (Mattson, 2002). At the time this study was conducted, first line oral medication (for example, fingolimod (Gilenya)) was available in the Netherlands on open trial basis. ABCNR medicines are injectable and self-administered. The clinical efficacy of DMT's – they reduce the number and severity of attacks and prolong the onset of secondary progressive MS – has been demonstrated in clinical trials however individual patients can continue to experience disease activity (Michel et al., 2015). In addition patients may experience side effects such as injection site reactions, flu-like symptoms, depression and arthritis (Michel et al., 2015). This increases the complexity in decision making for DMT's. Several studies report on the relatively low percentage of patients who act in accordance with the prescribed timing, dosing and frequency of medication (Evans et al., 2016; Hansen et al., 2015; Miller & Rhoades, 2012).

There are two strategies for treatment with DMT's in MS: therapeutic escalation or induction therapy (Michel et al., 2015). The idea behind therapeutic escalation is that treatment has to start with those medicines considered safest, before moving to more aggressive therapies. In induction therapy, the risk of rapidly progressive and definitive disability outweighs that of the adverse effects associated with the aggressive therapies. The decision for a specific treatment strategy is informed by the disease activity, burden of the disease, profile of adverse events, and also the patient's preference and the neurologist's experience (Michel et al., 2015). The studies included in the systematic review of Michel et al., show that disease activity, burden of disease, and the profile of adverse effects in relation to the use of DMT's have been studied intensively; however patients perspectives and neurologist experiences as factors in decision-making on DMT's for MS are under-researched. In this article we address this gap by conducting an explorative study about patient perspectives on the process of decision-making on DMT's for MS. The small body of literature that focuses on the patient perspective covers the point of decision-making (Johnson et al., 2006; Lowden, Lee, & Ritchie, 2014) and the user experience of DMT's (Miller & Jezewski, 2006; Miller, Karpinski, & Jezewski, 2012; Miller & Jezewski, 2001; Visser & Zande, 2011). Using DMT's is a lifelong affair. It is usually soon after the diagnosis of MS that patients are asked by their physicians to begin DMT's. Various qualitative studies have shown that the onset of the disease is characterized by experiences of uncertainty, loss, and grief (Dennison, Smith, Bradbury, & Galea, 2016; Dennison, Yardley, Devereux, & Moss-Morris, 2010; Miller, 1997). In addition to issues of getting used to the idea of having a chronic illness and exploring its meaning to their daily lives, patients are also faced with important decisions about DMT's. In this paper we set out to explore the perspectives of people with recently diagnoses MS on using DMT's.

Methodology

Design This study is part of the doctoral research project "Lived Experiences of People with Recently Diagnosed Multiple Sclerosis". The aim of this project is to examine the lived experiences of people with MS and the meaning of their diagnosis to their daily lives. It covers the themes of receiving the diagnosis (De Ceuninck van Capelle et al., 2016a), work (De Ceuninck van Capelle et al., 2015) and the meaning of MS within the context of family life (De Ceuninck van Capelle et al., 2016b). The study followed a phenomenological research design guided by Interpretative Phenomenological Analysis (IPA). IPA is a qualitative research approach committed to the examination of how people make sense of major life experiences (Smith et al., 2009). Since IPA studies are concerned with detailed examinations of particular cases they usually comprise a small number of participants. We used purposeful sampling to include people with a MS diagnosis according to the revised McDonald criteria (Polman et al., 2011) who had received their diagnosis no more than two years prior. Recruitment was carried out by a member of the interview team.[2] She called patients from the records of a hospital's ambulatory MS care to invite them to participate in our study. Recruitment was stopped when the number of participants had reached ten. The ethical committee of the St. Elisabeth Hospital in Tilburg approved the research and the patients gave informed consent to participation.

Data collection and Participants Because we were interested in how people make sense of the diagnosis in their daily life we opted for semi-structured interviews. This method allows the subjects the opportunity to tell their stories and to develop their ideas and express their concerns at length. Also, it enables the researcher and participant to engage in a dialogue whereby initial questions are modified in the light of participants' responses, and the researcher is able to pursue additional topics as they naturally emerge. The topic list used included the meaning of work, personal situation, diagnosis, and professional care. Although the recommendation to start DMT's was not on this topic list, it emerged as an important subject in the patient perspective as every participant mentioned it, whether they followed treatment or not. Consequently, we decided to add this theme to our study. The interviews were conducted by the first and the third author and a resident neurologist at the homes of the participants.

Data was gathered from 13 people: ten people with MS and three partners that were asked by the person with MS to assist them with the interviews. The interviews lasted at least one hour and up to more than two hours. All participants resided in the Netherlands and the patients and the participating partners were Caucasian. The participants with MS were aged 27-51 years. Table 1 shows the profile of the participants, ordered by age.

Table 1: Profile of the Participants

Participant	Interviewer	Gender	Age	No DMT's	DMT's	
					Injectable	Tablet
6	1st author	F	27		interferon beta 1a	
3	DF[3]	F	30		glatiramer acetate	

---

[2] DF, see Table 1.

[3] Daphne Frijlink MD.

46

9	1st author	F	31	V		
1	1st author	F	33	V		
5	1st author	M	35		glatiramer acetate	
10	1st author	F	41		interferon beta 1a	
8	3th author	F	43			fingolimod
7	3th author	F	45	V		
2	DF	M	46		glatiramer acetate	
4	DF	F	51		interferon beta 1a	

Data analysis Data analysis in IPA involves a double hermeneutic because the researcher makes sense of the participant trying to make sense of what is happening to them. The analysis can be understood as an iterative and multi-directional process involving description, interpretation, processes of reduction, flexible thinking, revision, creativity, and innovation. Most IPA studies follow a step-by-step approach in order to be systematic and rigorous, but these steps are always combined with an open attitude by the researchers. In this study, data analysis consisted of three stages of inductive analysis of the transcriptions. In the first stage, shortly after each interview, the authors and a postdoctoral researcher, independently from each other, added preparatory notes in Dutch in the right margins of the transcripts. Subsequently, the transcripts and notes were discussed in a plenary meeting. The cycle of interviewing, notating and discussing was repeated after each interview until the entire sample of ten interviews was completed. In the second stage, the first author systematized the notes from the first stage into a network of in vivo codes, supported by the data analysis software Atlas.ti version 6.2, using a constant comparison method. In the third stage, the first author used the network of codes to reconstruct a representation of patient perspectives on DMT's in four themes. The first author made a preliminary translation of the essential quotes falling under each theme. This translation was afterwards discussed and refined with the help of a professional translator (Van Nes, Abma, Jonsson, & Deeg, 2010).

Results

The analysis resulted in the identification of 4 interrelated themes: (1) Constant confrontation with the disease, (2) Managing inevitable decline, (3) Hope for improvement, and (4) Taking DMT's as a social experience. Table 2 shows by which codes from which transcripts the themes are supported. This table also shows the number of related units of experience (quotes) that support each code.

Table 2: Occurrence of themes in the transcripts

4 themes, supporting codes in each transcript and number of quotes included in each code	Pharmacological situation		
	No DMT's	Injectable	Tablet
(1) Constant confrontation with the disease	P1, P9	P2, P3, P6, P10	
P1: situation 11 (6[4])			
P2: pain (5), medication (6), body (11)			
P3: injecting (9)			
P6: pushing the button (3), injecting (6), fear (9), medication (11			
P9: new medication (1), pricking (3), injecting (4), fear (12)			
P10: denial (3), acceptance (4), declining treatment (4), injecting (10)			
(2) Managing inevitable decline	P7	P4, P5, P10	
P4: abandoning injecting (1), injecting (3), medication (4)			
P5: hope (3), medication (5)			
P7: medication (4)			
P10: denial (3), acceptance (4), declining treatment (4), injecting (10)			
(3) Hope for improvement		P4, P10	P8
P4: abandoning injecting (1), injecting (3), medication (4)			
P8: linking perceived progress with treatment (1), taking tablets (3), experimental treatment (11)			
P10: denial (3), acceptance (4), declining treatment (4), injecting (10)			
(4) Taking DMT's as a social experience		P2, P5, P6, P10	P8
P2: pain (5), medication (6), body (11)			
P5: hope (3), medication (5)			
P6: pushing the button (3), injecting (6), fear (9), medication (11)			
P8: linking perceived progress with treatment (1), taking tablets (3), experimental treatment (11)			
P10: denial (3), acceptance (4), declining treatment (4), injecting (10)			

---

[4] This code name refers to P1's reflections about starting treatment with injectable medicine.

Constant confrontation with the disease. All participants felt caught off guard by the recommendation to begin DMT's. This feeling was related with the mode of administration (usually injections) and / or the prospect of having to use medication with possible side-effects for the rest of their lives. Three participants (P3 (using an injectable), P8 (taking tablets) and P9 (not using immunomodulating medication)) expressed interesting and similar feelings about using an injectable in contrast to taking a pill. The idea of taking injections (initially) scared them. The meanings behind this fear seem to vary. Some participants told how initially they struggled to find good 'spots' for injecting medicines and to 'view' their bodies from the (technical) angle of injecting medicines. P2 told in detail how he had learned with the help of his wife to operate the injection device. P3 and P8 welcomed oral administration (through pills) as a – in contrast to injections – much more 'natural' way to take medicines. Rather than operational and technical causes of fear, they raised emotional and relational ones. The idea of taking injections (initially) made them to feel distanced from others, while with pills it was felt possible to preserve a degree of normalcy. *"Pills, well, everybody sometimes takes a pill, a vitamin pill. But this is different. You have to inject yourself. The first time I was really shocked that I had to do this. But once the needle was in [my body], I felt relief. After that I started to experiment a bit. Now, injecting [medicine] is okay with me."* {P3:295}

Besides ponderings bout the mode of administration, the prospect of having to use heavy medication for the rest of their lives also surfaced as an element of continuous confrontation with disease. P1 felt a 'barrier' to starting medication. This barrier had in her perception partially to do with not knowing how to weigh possible risks (occurrence of side effects) against possible benefits (delay of progression). The wish to become pregnant was felt by P1 as an opportunity to set aside this matter for another time (taking medication during pregnancy is discouraged). For another participant (P8), a quite 'literal' barrier surfaced in that having started medication she at first no longer felt safe to travel long distances (in Europe), away from her own hospital where professionals knew her and her medication. Confrontation with disease meant for her and other participants the confrontation with a world that looked less navigable and less free. Participant 10 phrased her feeling of illness and medicines imposing limitations on her life as follows: *"[The moment that] the doctor proposed to begin medication I thought: 'If I start, there will be no way back. In that case, I head straight towards acknowledging the fact that my life and my body are leaving me behind.'"* {P10:33}

Managing inevitable decline. The recommendation sparked either an affirmative or negative response from the participants. Like table 1 shows, at the time of the interview, 7 of the 10 participants used medication. All participants said that they had been actively engaged with a decision about medication. Some of them perceived the limited chance to delay progression as at least *one* opportunity to do something about their situation. *"[My doctor] gave me tablets to suppress my shakiness. And then he proposed starting me on injections. I replied: 'If it helps, I consent to anything!' So I started injecting the medication. I don't have any problem with that, with doing injections."* {P4:78} But one other participant, P7, perceived the limited efficacy of medication not as an opportunity for delay of progress of illness in her life, but rather as a sign of a poor product. *"Even if the efficacy had been just fifty percent, the choice [in favor of treatment] would have been easier. But it is just thirty percent. The efficacy of a placebo is thirty percent as well. That makes me think: 'I'll take a Smartie instead.' (...) Thirty percent, that is so little."* {P7:144} Lived expectations for efficacy of medicines to manage inevitable decline hence varied through the sample. Most participants hoped to be part of the lucky 30%, for whom using medicines has a positive effect.

Hope for improvement. The participants that followed the recommendation to start treatment hoped that adherence to treatment would be effective in slowing down the progression of the disease. But the sample indicates that 'hope' refers to more than just the statistical information about the efficacy of medicines during the entire lifespan of a patient that is part of a representative population of patients.

First, hope is also connected with perceived physical conditions *here* and *now*. Participants felt motivated to continue treatment when they felt good. In the same manner some of them felt disappointed when 'despite' taking medication, they went through a relapse. A fragment that illustrates how statistical and experiential knowledge about medicines can contrast with each other is as follows: *"But then, the strength of my left leg began to fade. (...) I told him [my doctor]: 'I want to stop with injections". He replied: 'Yes, there is only a thirty percent chance that the medication will keep you stable'. And yes, I remembered that he told me that before. But once my legs and my awareness began to be affected, I began to despair. 'Why do I keep going on with injections? It doesn't help me anyway.'"* {P4:93}.

Second, besides being connected to the perceived physical condition *here* and *now*, 'hope' had in our sample also a relational dimension. An oral medication, Gilenya (Fingolimod), that at the time of the interview was not yet covered by health insurances in the Netherlands, had become for participant 8 an object that signified how she worked together with her family against her disease: *"And even my family said – The medicine costs 65 euros each day, so that's 25000 euros each year – last Easter: 'We don't know how we will raise the money to pay for those medicines, but we will find a way to pay for it, if necessary we will pay it ourselves.' I'm really lucky to be surrounded by such people. And that gives me hope, every time."* {8:179} Clearly in this fragment it is not only the expected efficacy of the medicine that gives the participant hope. Her hope is also related to the proximity of her family. They support her in living with her disease. By paying for her medicine (or the willingness to do so if necessary), they stay with her. She's not left on her own.

Taking DMT's as a social experience. Taking or declining to take medicines was for all participants a social experience. Consideration of adhering to treatment was something that was discussed with family and friends before participants made a decision. After the decision to start treatment, family and also the MS nurse (either from the hospital or from the manufacturer of the medicine), continued to appear as important elements in the lived experience of using medicines: *"In the beginning, injecting myself caused me a lot of pain. I have an automatic injection pen. It is adjustable from 0 to 10. But I had absolutely no clue how the button worked. So after a month, I called [MS nurse] Lisa, because I had a couple of times injected my leg like this and the needle penetrated my leg very deeply. (...) Lisa explained to me how to modify the injection pen with the button and adjust it to level 4 or 6. So now I use level 4 for my legs and level 6 for my stomach, because then you can inject with more force."* {P2:143} Other participants explained how their contact with the MS nurse from the manufacturer went beyond the technicalities of administration. They felt the call from the nurse as an opportunity to get their concerns about having MS of their chest. Participant 6 told how she had become depended on her father and boyfriend to take her medication: *"That medication [interferon beta 1a] has to be administered by injection. In the beginning I did this myself; the MS nurse explained to me how I had to do it. I was very scared and felt very nervous about it. Actually, I still do. I [even] don't dare to do it [injecting] myself anymore."* {P6:121} In this and a few other fragments, taking medicines presents itself as a mode wherein relationships with close others (father, boyfriend, spouse) are lived.

Discussion

The clearest finding to emerge from the analysis is that, in the patient's perspective, dealing with the advice to start treatment with DMT's is a highly complicated phenomenon. Participants struggled to form personal understandings about statistical information on medical benefits and risks, and felt scared about administering injections. Once treatment had started, fear of injections and doubts about efficacy reappeared in some participants, but most of them managed to make treatment with DMT's part of their normal daily life. The observed complexity of decision making, adjustment and adherence corroborates the findings of previous studies (Johnson et al., 2006; Lowden et al., 2014; Miller & Jezewski, 2006; Miller & Jezewski, 2001).

In an attempt to define the core issue behind decision making on DMT's in MS, Lowden et al. (2014) proposed understanding it as the redefinition of the self. (Lowden et al., 2014). We think that the themes "Constant confrontation with the disease" and "Managing inevitable decline" align with this explanation. At the outset, the injection pen presented itself to some participants as an alien device that was difficult to control. Yet, over time, participants 'allowed' MS and the injection pen to become a part of their normal life, abandoning the pessimistic images and, guided by their own day to day experiences, developed, a more balanced perspective. This is in line with the understanding of DMT's in MS as a matter of the redefinition of the self. Yet, the remaining two themes, "Hope for improvement" and "Taking DMT's as a social experience" line up less well with redefinition of the self as the way how patients view the process of adapting to DMT's in MS. The presence of supportive others and the presence of hope are not just matters of individual development. Rather they emphasize the relevance of meaningful relationships and the need for a livable future to decision-making on and adherence to medication. Consequently, we think that redefinition of the self needs to be complemented by hope and the proximity of supportive others as two other essential elements in the patient perspective on decision-making on and use of DMT's in MS.

Perhaps the most intriguing finding indeed is the use DMT's as a social experience. Five of the seven participants explained that using DMT's was, for them, a strongly relational experience, either because of practical or financial support from family members, or because of good relations with the hospital staff and the nurses from pharmaceutical industry-sponsored patient support programs. And one of the three participants (P7) who didn't use medicines at the time of the interview also indicated during the interview that her decision *not* to take medicines had been thoroughly discussed with her family and partner. This finding corroborates the studies of Johnson et al. (2006), Miller & Jezewski (2001) and Miller & Jezewski (2006) and Lowden et al. (2014), who also found the support of others as a theme in decision making and administration of DMT's. In this century, health *information* technology has become an established practice and field of research. Strongly connected with the rise of this field of research is the idea that medical decision making is (foremost) rational and the result of interaction between individuals. But our small study about DMT's as lived phenomena within the lifeworld of patients shows a different picture. People not only think about medication, but also have feelings about it. The role of relationships that provide for the social framework wherein communication in health care flows is largely an area that remains to be explored. Future research should address this gap.

We found in qualitative research literature very little on the question of why patients discontinue DMT's while it often occurs in practice. The only previous study that has included the perspectives of patients (n=2) about stopping DMT's is Johnson et al. (2006). In our study, just one participant (P4) had considered discontinuing because of disappointment about the efficacy of DMT's. This adds up to the reasons why patients give up of adherence to DMT's, besides problems with self-injection and not feeling ill enough to justify treatment, that surfaced in the study of Johnson et al. (2006) as to other reasons for stopping. Given the estimation that the adherence rate in injectable DMT's is sometimes as high as 49% (Menzin et al., 2012), we think that patient perspectives on discontinuation of adherence is an important issue for future research.

Several limitations to this study need to be acknowledged. Since the only inclusion criterion was time span between diagnosis and day of the interview, we included participants in dissimilar pharmacological situations. This allowed us to explore diverse ways of dealing with the use of DMT's. But it disadvantaged any deeper investigation of the meaning of specific DMT's. Investigation of specific DMT's as a phenomenon would be a fruitful direction for future research. Another limitation we note is that the stories of the participants reflect, generally, a situation of stability in disease course and medication use. Future studies should address adverse events (Brandes, Callender, Lathi, & O'Leary, 2008), unexpected progression of disease course, treatment failure and switching to other DMT's as subjects of research in the patient perspective on using DMT's in MS.

Excursus: Participant #10 on starting with DMT's

"I want to be looked after by *him* because with him I feel free to ask whatever I want."

"A year [after the disclosure of the diagnosis] they advised me:
'OK. It would be a good idea to start treatment.'
But I thought:
'Why? I don't understand.'
But he [the neurologist that had also told me my diagnosis] couldn't explain to me what motivated him to advise me to start treatment. So I thought by myself:
'Shit, that's you stuck in the process of acceptance.'
But then my sister in law said:
'Why don't you go talk with Dr. Farjadi? You know, getting another point of view, taking a different angle …'
So that's what I did.
Once engaged in conversation [with him] I felt:
'Yes, this is what I call good information, I feel conformable to ask whatever I want, without worrying myself about … hmm.'
I thought:
'Yes I like this a lot more.'
Strange, but instantly I felt:
'Yes, but in that case I want to switch. I don't want treatment. But if I have to return to the hospital at a regular basis anyway – I have an incurable disease, they can't heal me – I want to be looked after by Dr. Farjadi. He gives good explanations and with him I feel free to ask whatever I want.' [P10-112-117]"[5]

The previously introduced distinction between the "biomedical voice" and "the voice of experience" (Toombs 1988, Frank 2000) may well serve here also as a point of departure for reflection. In the account of participant #10 (Renata), the biomedical voice surfaces in the presentation of starting treatment as a "good idea" (Costello et al., 2016), in the psychological concepts of "acceptance" and "denial" (Dennison et al., 2010) and, finally, in the prerogative of medical information (at the expense of experience and emotion as complementary sources of knowledge) in the medical encounter (Krahn 2013, Elian 1985). The "voice of experience" is also present. It emerges first in the rather vague initial resistance to accept treatment (Renata herself struggles to understand this resistance of hers). Also it emerges in the discovery that in the second setting with the other neurologist Renata doesn't feel her person and the range of her questions in danger to be limited. In the acquaintance of Renata with Dr. Farjadi the "voice of medicine" and the "voice of experience" come together and shape a track that Renata's feels to be able to follow.

---

[5] Shortly after her switch participant #10 started with DMT.

The "voice of experience" in dealing with DMT's may well serve to enhance and to bring to life the biomedical concept of adherence. "Adherence" is defined by the World Health Organization as "the extent to which a person's behavior – taking medication, following a diet, and/or executing lifestyle changes – corresponds with agreed upon recommendations from a health care provider." (Sabate 2003). According to this definition the fragment above can be read as an account of the initial refusal of Renata to agree with the recommendation of her healthcare provider (the first neurologist) to start DMT's. But the fragment clearly shows that there is more to say about dealing with DMT's than the concepts "agreement" and "recommendation" capture. To use the expression 'agreement' curtails the apprehension of what shows itself. There is something different at stake. DMT's as a phenomenon signifies for Renata the irreversible entrance illness in her regular life for the rest of her life and this perspective troubles her. In the words of Toombs the start with DMT's may affect the principal openness of Renata's *life project* towards the future since now it will be always a be future of which the regular use of DMT's will be a defining characteristic (Toombs 1988). Agreement to use of DMT's is therefore not just sticking to what the doctor says. It requires from the patient the development of a completely new outlook on his or her present and future. This implies that support for persons that consider DMT's might need to entail a lot more than the usual information about benefits and risks of treatment.

The lesson that we learn from the previous chapter is that long term therapies (with drugs) are as much the domain of the patient as a person that of the physician. Adherence to DMT's as a phenomenon is *not* just about showing behavior that corresponds with recommendations that were previously agreed on. This concept of "adherence" only represents the "voice of medicine" and is therefore in want of completion. As a phenomenon in the lifeworld of the patient DMT's signify the introduction of the challenge to bring the life project in line with a disease that is varying, incurable and difficult to predict. The case of Renata shows that a patient may not passively wait until providers of care have created an environment in which the conditions for an acceptable (from the perspective of the patient) application of DMT's can be met. Rather, she actively searches and finds an environment that provides a safe haven for her person and her worries about DMT's and receiving long term care. We propose here the idea that change of care providers, the very existence of 'complementary' and 'alternative' medicine in MS (Yadav et al., 2014), the occurrence of questionable (and expensive) requests for of second opinions and tests, point to the failure of mainstream medicine to *combine* skillful application of scientific technology with the cultivation (Toombs 2001) of a professional habit of mind (Greenfield 2010) that is aware of illness and care such as they are lived by the patient.

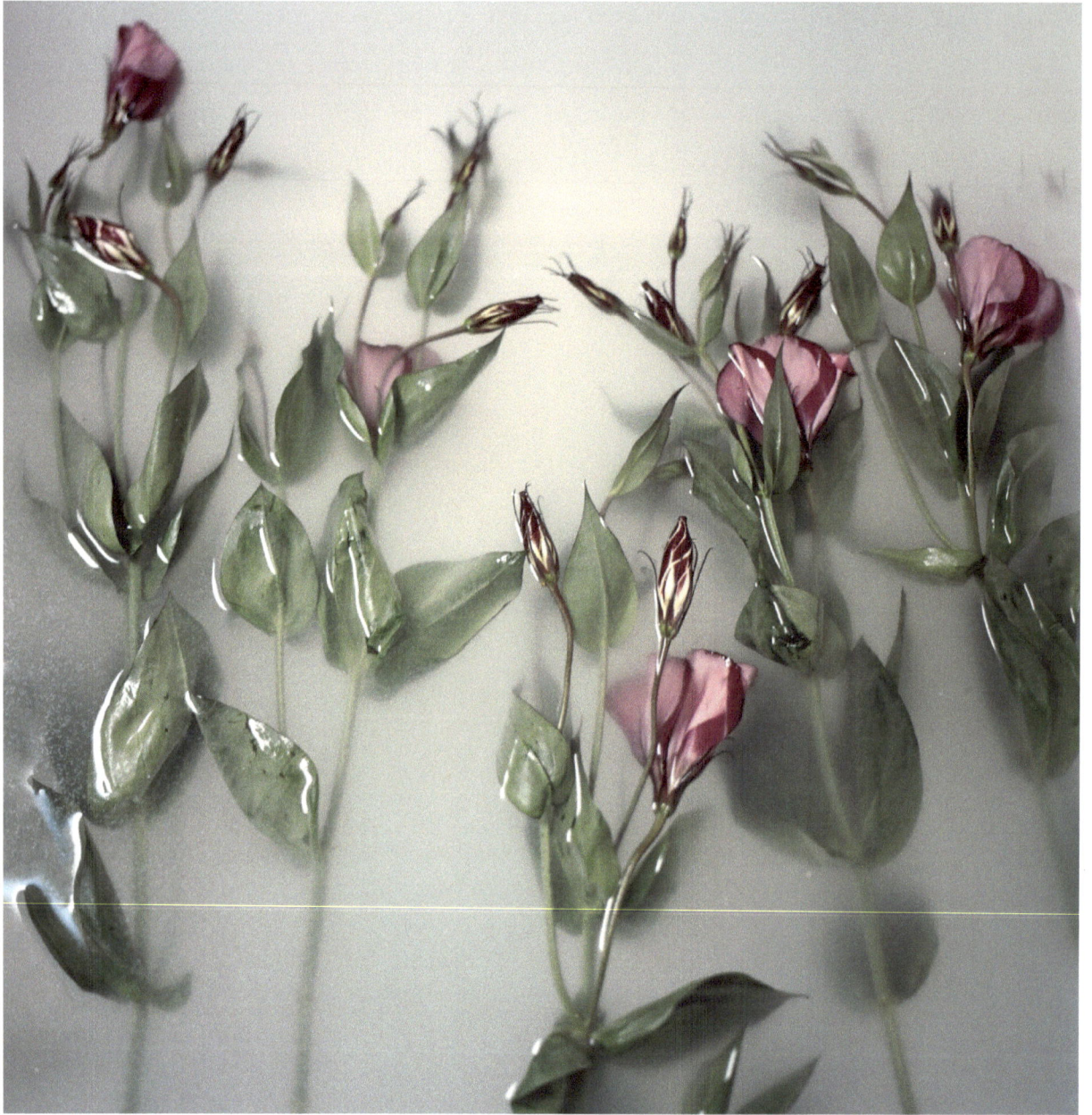

3. MS AS A FAMILY ISSUE

Introduction: In this study the authors explored how people with recently diagnosed multiple sclerosis (MS) experience their disease within their family lives. Ten people in various stages of the cycle of family life (leaving home, finding a partner, raising children, parenting adolescents, launching children) who had been diagnosed with MS were interviewed in half-structured conversational interviews. Method: Transcriptions were analyzed following a phenomenological approach. Results: Five themes were found: (a) dwindling capacity for housekeeping and childcare (b) struggling to ask for or to accept help, (c) countering awkward attitudes toward my illness, (d) suspecting family members of concealing their feelings, and (e) watching family members wrestle with your illness. Discussion: The participants described that their illness affected their ability to care for their family and home as they used to. Only a couple of studies have addressed the first person perspective of patients on family and MS. The study expands on these studies by exploring not previously examined perspectives on leaving home, finding a partner, parenting adolescents, and launching children. The findings on family and MS, approached as elements of the first person perspective of MS patients, may guide future research. Given the pivotal role of worries on family in patient experience of MS, we argue that acknowledgment of family as a constitutive element of the patient perspective should be integrated in regular MS care. The authors suggest that the clinical handling of MS as a family issue needs to be done thoughtfully and with attention to the specificities of each unique family situation.

Keywords: Multiple Sclerosis, qualitative research, first person perspectives, stages of the cycle of family life, care

Ceuninck van Capelle, A. de, Visser, L. H., & Vosman, F. J. H. (2016). Multiple Sclerosis (MS) in the Life Cycle of the Family: An Interpretative Phenomenological Analysis of the Perspective of Persons With Recently Diagnosed MS. Families, Systems, & Health. Advance online publication. doi: 10.1037/fsh0000216

Introduction

Multiple sclerosis (MS) is a chronic, and sometimes progressive neurological illness. There is no cure for MS, but disease-modifying therapies are available. Treatment of MS has followed the transition in Western health care from physician centered to patient- and family-centered care. Currently, self-management by the patient and family, patient and family education, and the patient's and family's quality of life are considered to be pivotal elements in what is called comprehensive care in MS (Halper, 2008). Previous studies, assessing the effects of couple- and family-based interventions in the treatment of various common diseases, have showed that such interventions may have small but promising effects on health outcome for both the patient and his or her family (Hartmann, Bäzner, Wild, Eisler, & Herzog, 2010; Shields, Finley, Chawla, & others, 2012). A causal approach to family-based care in MS that focusses at effects of interventions would be valuable and remains to be done, however in this paper we have taken a different angle and have studied family and MS as elements of the patient experience of illness. Even though family as an element of the patient experience of illness is a familiar phenomenon for clinicians, only a very small number of studies excavate family and illness as parts of the patient perspective (Audulv, Packer, & Versnel, 2014). Finlay (2003) described in her study the lifeworld of a young mother, analyzing her experience of living with early stage MS as the inter-twining of self, body, and world. Payne & McPherson (2010) explored strategies of women and their families for mothering young children while living with MS. In this article we expand on these studies by focusing specifically at the first persons perspective of the patient within the first 2 years after the making of the definitive diagnosis relapsing remitting MS.

Method

The design of the study, data collection, number of participants, data analysis follow the guide-lines of interpretative phenomenological analysis (Smith et al., 2009) and have been described in detail in a recent publication (De Ceuninck van Capelle et al., 2015). Data were gathered from 10 people with a definitive relapsing remitting MS diagnosis who had received their diagnosis within the last 2 years. Three participants asked the researchers for permission to be accompanied by their partner during the interview. We granted this request. The interviews were guided by a 4-point topic list, addressing diagnosis, work, private life, and medical care. The analysis was supported by software package ATLAS.ti, version 6.1. All participants were residents of the Netherlands, Caucasian, and aged 27–51 years. Table 1 shows the profile of the participants.

Table 1: Profile of the participants

Participant	Interviewer[6]	Gender[7]	Age	Partner?	Household composition participant
6	1st author	F	27	yes	living alone
3	DF	F	30	no	living alone
9	1st author	F	31	yes	couple, toddler
1	1st author	F	33	yes	couple
5	1st author	M	35	yes*	couple, school aged children
10	1st author	F	41	yes	couple, school aged children
8	2nd author	F	43	yes	couple, adolescent children
7	2nd author	F	45	yes	couple, school aged and adolescent children
2	DF	M	46	yes*	couple, adult disabled daughter
4	DF	F	51	yes*	chronically ill couple, adult daughter

* Partner present at the interview at the request of the participant

Data analysis consisted of three stages. In the first stage, shortly after each interview, the authors and a postdoc researcher added, independently from each other, preparatory notes in the right-hand margins of the audio transcriptions. Subsequently the annotated transcriptions were discussed in a plenary meeting. The cycle of interviewing, noting, and discussing was repeated each time until the entire sample of 10 interviews was finished. In the second stage, Archie de Ceuninck van Capelle approached the transcriptions as sources for the exploration of first person

---

[6] DF = Daphne Frijlink MD, see acknowledgements.
[7] M = Male, F= Female.

experiences. He coded in vivo akin units of experience with names referring to the content of each unit. Units were sometimes coded with several codes because of overlapping content. In the third, concluding stage, Archie de Ceuninck van Capelle compared, in close collaboration with Leo H. Visser and Frans J. H. Vosman, the coded units of experience with the initial interview topics. They found the topic "private life" associated with five intersecting clusters of units of experience. Also these clusters appeared to traverse with phases in the cycle of family life.

Results

We refer to the content of the clusters of units of experience as follows: (a) dwindling capacity for housekeeping and care, (b) struggling to ask for or to accept help, (c) countering awkward attitudes toward my illness, (d) suspecting family members to conceal feelings, and (e) watching family members wrestle with your illness. Table 2 shows by which codes from which transcriptions the themes are supported. This table shows also the number of akin units of experience (quotes) that supports each code. Table 3 displays for each theme two typical quotes and the names with which these quotes where coded.

Table 2: Occurrence of themes in the transcriptions

5 themes, supporting codes in each transcription and number of quotes included in each code	Phase in the cycle of family life[8]		
	starting	realizing	finishing
(1) dwindling capacity for housekeeping and care	P1[9], P5,	P7, P8,	P4
P1: getting things done (3), experiencing limitations (4), desire for offspring (4), fatigue (7)	PP5[10],	P10	
P4: daughter is suspected to restrain herself (2), marriage (2), dwindling capacities (7), fatigue (15), impact on the family (16)	P9		
P5: planning ahead is difficult (1), sight (7)			
PP5: desire for offspring (4), cognitive impairments (6)			
P7: walking with children (5), explaining impairment to children (5), holidays (5), being a mom (6), my daughter (7), my son (7), counting with your limitations (8), childcare (9), my partner (10)			

---

[8] Phases according to the model of the cycle of family life of Carter and McGoldrick, cited in Rolland (2005).
[9] Participant #1.
[10] Partner of participant #5.

P8: dishwasher (2), experiencing limitations (3), daughter (4), children take illness into account (4), father (6), grief (6), children growing into teenagers (9), sight (10), home (10), family (13), fatigue (16), children (21), mother (25), partner (26)			
P9: family (2), not avoiding breaks anymore (2), childcare requires strength (2), family planning (4), cleaning (4), being a mom (5), need for making adaptations (5), personal standards for housekeeping (6), daughter (10), fatigue (11), house (13)			
P10: telling your limits (2), house (3), father (3), fatigue (5), adapting to MS (7), scheduling breaks (7), children (8), mother (14)			
(2) wrestling to ask for or to accept help	P1, PP5	P8, P10	P2, P4
P1: what occupies me (7) getting things done (3), experiencing limitations (4), fatigue (7)			
P2: dependency (3)			
P4: grief (2), feeling forced to give up responsibilities (9), concentration and memory (15)			
PP5: I have learned to ask for help (3)			
P8: victory (2), allowing to be looked after (3), wrestling to accept help (7), partner (26)			
P10: learning to accept help (2), accepting offers of help (3)			
(3) fighting awkward attitudes towards illness	P1, P3, P6	P7	
P1: annoying attitudes (5)			
P3: people think that I'm lazy (9), people must know about my MS (12), feeling (not) understood (13), people are scared of MS (16), feeling perceived as a weak person (16), incomprehension (17), people don't understand MS (20)			
P6: feeling awkward (2), my boyfriend's mother (3), being patronized (4), feeling exposed (8), feeling vulnerable (11), they don't know how to take a stance (13), first period (16), unfamiliarity (18)			
P7 public identity as a patient (3)			
(4) suspecting family members to conceal feelings		P8, P10	P4
P4: daughter is suspected to restrain herself (2)			
P8: daughter (4), children (21)			
P10: house (3), fatigue (5) observing me and drawing private conclusions (6), my life (7), mother (14)			
(5) watching family members wrestling with your illness	P3, P5, PP5, P6, P9,	P8, P7, P9	
P3: mother (13), grief (10)			
P5: parents (3), toddler (1)			
PP5: toddler (1)			
P6: boyfriend is scared of MS (4), is my boyfriend able to talk (4), friends (8), father (12), boyfriend (15)			
P7: father (4), brothers (4), silence about MS in the family (14)			

P8: attention from the neighbourhood (3), father (6), friends (6), mother (25)			
P9: partner (12)			

Table 3: Typical quotes for each theme

Theme	Quotation [participant #: quotation #]	Code(s)[11]
(1)	[P9:139] "Yes, I have become more relaxed. Now I think: 'Okay, some toys have been dropped here, but too bad; I leave them there and just pass them by. Shortly [after her afternoon nap], she [my daughter] will be downstairs again and once more it will be a mess.' But in the past, I was cleaning up every five minutes. But that's over now. I'm not doing it anymore. Period.	need for making adaptations (5), daughter (10), house (13)
	[P8:246] "Now, my husband is emptying the dishwasher. In the past however, I refused him to do that. At home, *I* was the person that supervised everything. Yes, I did it all, I cared well. Admitting that [I had MS and needed help] was quite a victory."	dishwasher (2), home (10), partner (26)
(2)	[P1:51] "Now, I have the courage to ask for help. (…) At first it was a big step for me to call for help, I used to be very self-reliant. But now I just need to ask for help, and yes, all this is part of the deal [of living with MS].	getting things done (3), experiencing limitations (4), fatigue (7)
	[P4:85-86] Not being self-reliant anymore, having to leave things to someone else, that's very difficult for me. Even when it is the doctor or my husband. My husband has a lot on his mind, he's ill, like me [*eyes of the participant water*]. I used to take care of him, after I had returned from work."	grief (2), feeling forced to give up responsibilities (9)
(3)	[P6:53] "The mother of my boyfriend – she works in the hospital as a nurse, formerly at the emergency care unit – told me: 'Yeah, every part of your body fails, finally your heart too, and then ….you know!' So everybody started [after I had received my diagnosis] to 'inform' me about what was going happen to me."	feeling awkward (2), my boyfriend's mother (3), being patronized (4), feeling exposed (8), feeling vulnerable (11), they don't know how to take a stance (13), first period (16), unfamiliarity (18)
	[P3:27] "I don't like it at all when people [say or think]: 'She's so pitiful' or something like that."	people must know about my MS (12), feeling (not) understood (13), people

---

[11] Code name(s) and number of quotes included in each code.

		are scared of MS (16), feeling perceived as a weak person (16)
(4)	[P4:113-114] "And she [my adult daughter] kept things hidden from me. When she was preoccupied with a problem, she would think: 'Mama forgets it', or, 'Mama is already occupied enough, so I won't tell her.' So ... [one day] I took her by her arm and put her on the couch and said: 'Now we talk! You just tell me everything, in a calm way, and hide nothing. Despite my MS, I want you to tell me everything!'"	daughter is suspected to restrain herself (2)
	[P8:215] "Often when she [my daughter] is elsewhere [visiting someone], they [the hosts] ask: 'How is [your] mom doing? In this way they [son and daughter] are affected by it [my illness], but you [I] never hear about that."	daughter (4), children (21)
(5)	[P3:124-126] "When I talk about my complaints, yes, I hear her ... eh ... swallow. – *Interviewer: What do you notice?* – Lots of grief. And I think that it will never leave her."	mother (13), grief (10)
	[P6:26] "It [my illness] weighs on him [my boyfriend] a lot. But he can't talk about it [with me]."	is my boyfriend able to talk (4), boyfriend (15)

The themes can be summarized as follows. (a) Most participants cared proudly for others (children, partner, parents) and were in charge of their households at the time that MS started to affect their family lives. Fatigue and cognitive problems were felt to interfere severely with their ability to care. (b) Some participants outlined "help" as a theme of its own. Accepting help from mother or partner meant for them consequently their illness and limitations becoming more real. (c) A couple of participants highlighted awkward attitudes (including well-meant "offers" for help) toward their illness, overstating their position as a patient, misapprehending symptoms and spreading ignorance about MS without even knowing it. (d) MS felt for four participants to spoil emotional intimacy between them and their children or mother. The lost harmony in the family was experienced in feelings of distance and isolation. (e) What most participants saw of the feelings and thoughts of their family members was not very encouraging: fear, grief and confusion.

Discussion

The participants living with recently diagnosed MS described that their illness affected the way they used to be able to care for their family and home. They noticed, in conversations with close relatives, under- as well as overemphasis on the role of illness in their daily lives. Both attitudes were viewed as unwanted and annoying. Only a couple of previous studies have addressed the first person perspective of patients on family life and MS. Under- and overemphasis in MS was also observed by Grytten & Måseide (2006) who conceptualized this phenomenon as a matter of social stigma. Our study runs parallel with their symbolic interactionist account of stigma, whereas with a phenomenological approach we have been strictly concentrating on the first person's perspective, that of the patient: the social phenomenon of stigmatization provokes personal resistance against popular images of MS and stimulates the discovery of one's interpretation of illness. Dwindling capacity for care, growing need for help, and observed feelings of grief of those close to the patient show powerfully that MS is a phenomenon that affects family systems and not just individuals. This finding fits within the psychosocial typology of illness by Rolland (2005) and complements current research using this typology with a view of the specific interface of family and recently diagnosed MS. This interface is characterized by an unpredictable disease course and a mix of motor as well as cognitive impairments which can be temporary as well as permanent. Our findings corroborate with Payne & McPherson (2010) on mothering young children and add to this study by also including perspectives on care for adolescents and young adults. The unpredictable and sometimes progressive nature of MS made was reflected in our results especially by its perceived interference with the early phases in the cycle of family life. In these stages the nature of MS hastened the decision for a first pregnancy (to stay ahead of expected deterioration of health) or made participants to avoid a second or third pregnancy (to minimize the burden of raising a family while having MS).

We do note that this study has some limitations. Our method of data collection has resulted in the presence of various stages of the cycle of family life in the sample. This has allowed us to get an exploratory broad overview of the first person perspective of patients of MS on family life. But the study has not achieved saturation which would require a more focused sample. Another limitation is that stories of the participants reflected the overall situation of normal, day-to-day living with MS. Future research should examine more closely emergencies like relapses and ask how the developmental tasks associated with each stage in family life interfere with MS. Finally, all the family arrangements that are covered in this study are traditional. Future research should seek to also address other family types. Regarding the implications of this study for clinical practice, we estimate that the small number of studies that deal with MS and family as perspectival issues point out that the integration of the perspective of MS patients – including "family" as an element of this perspective – in MS care is still in its infancy. But, given the picture, arising also from this study, that in the patient experience of MS, the family theme seems to be pivotal, we hope that our study inspires clinicians to see and acknowledge the meaning of family for patients while providing care for families living with MS. Also our study indicates that family situations strongly vary. This suggests that the clinical handling of MS as a family issue needs to be done thoughtfully and with attention for the particulars of each family situation.

"If you only knew how tired I feel right now"

> I never want to lay down on the sofa [to rest]. I don't want them [my kids] to remember me like:
>
> 'Oh, well, when I [was young and] returned home from school my mother used to lay on the sofa.'
>
> No, I hate that so I prevent that. So if I lay myself down on the sofa I choose a position that enables me to see them when they come home. I don't want them to remember me like:
>
> 'Oh, mom was always so tired, she used to lay on the sofa.'
>
> I really don't want that. I don't want them to be affected by a bad memory [of me once they're adults]. But you know sometimes I feel so tired and then suddenly [my son] Luke pops up and says for example:
>
> 'Mom, can you give me something to drink?'
>
> And at such a moment I say:
>
> 'Fetch it yourself, Luke.'
>
> 'Well, oh, okay, pfff.'
>
> More often than not these kind of situations are resolved well. But sometimes I think:
>
> 'Please be considerate just for a second to the fact that I am so tired, if you only knew how tired I feel right now.'
>
> And that is the fight that we have between us. You want them and you don't want them to reckon with [the fact that I have MS]." [P8:208-210]

This study is outlined according to the second critical insight of the ethics of care that situatedness and contextuality need to be recognized (Klaver 2013). In the first two chapters we studied how people with MS experience illness and care in the context of professional care in MS. In the previous chapter we turned to a second context – the family – in which illness and care appear as phenomena of the patient experience of MS. As an analogue to our approach to care as a relational network we understand family as a framework wherein people can appear to each other as real persons. This implies that we adopt a non-romantic view of family relationships: family can be the space where people appear as they are and meet some acceptance for that. It does not imply nice, warm, non-antagonistic, all-accepting relationships. Next to our realistic description of family there are other characteristics, inspired by phenomenology: it is possible to get an initial phenomenological understanding of the family along the notions of time, space, and embodiment (Toombs 1988). Family as a phenomenon entails the distribution of time in generations and lifetimes. It entails moreover a specific organization of spaces and relationships (a household that consists of a single nuclear family with growing children). Finally the family as an embodied phenomenon involves the (gendered) distribution and organization of professional and domestic tasks and the maintenance of a sexual life. The arrangement of time, space and embodiment that constitutes the family as a horizon for human life can be disrupted (Toombs 1988) by the occurrence of a (medical) event like the onset of MS.

The fragment above shows a fine example of how such a disruption may evolve. Participant #8 (Savina) worries about how her children will remember her as a mother. This as such is a complicated form of awareness at the present time: to imagine how one will be seen later on, be remembered. The gaze of others, but also the gaze of others later on, makes up a complex dorm of awareness. It is not about what her children see now. Savina fears that her illness will cause her to be remembered later as a bad mother. A normal succession of generations in which children keep their parents in loving memory is thwarted. Disruption of space and embodiment is also evident in the fragment. Savina gives the example of her son Luke asking for a drink. Affected by a wave of fatigue (embodiment) she doesn't feel to be able to respond to the need of her child (relationship) by walking to the kitchen (space) to bring him his drink.

Disruption is moreover also discernible at the level of conditions that allow for a subject to appear as an ethical being and as the bearer of an ethical claim (Murray & Holmes 2014). We introduced this level of analysis in the first section of this study in the paragraph about our application of an adapted version of IPA. The ethical claim "But sometimes I think: 'Please be considerate just for a second to the fact that I am so tired, if you only knew how tired I feel right now'" is expressed in the fragment only in an *imagined* relational scene of address. Instead of telling her son the reason why she can't bring him his drink – disease-related fatigue – she hides it and just asks him get it himself. The fragment hence presents an instance of family as a framework wherein the person with MS might also *not* appear as the bearer of an ethical claim. The tension between the wish to make manifest the effects of disease (fatigue) and the desire to the prevent disease from ruining the prevailing organization of the family (including the way in which Savina wishes to be remembered as a mother) deteriorate in the example the conditions that are necessary to be seen as a person with MS. We do have a strong lead that imagination and the gaze of others are constituents of the phenomenality of lived experience. This may have big and practical implications for care givers: to not psychologize but to follow the trajectory of revelations of lived experience, also in its more advanced or even complex forms of imagination and taking into account the gaze of meaningful others.

Against the background of a phenomenological reading of the fragment of participant #8 we want to situate the previous chapter in the framework of our study by making two points. The first point refers to phenomenology as a moral approach to care. One might wonder what this exactly entails. In the introduction of this study we connected the idea of phenomenology as a moral approach to care with the exploration of the voice of experience as voice that communicates suffering (Toombs 1988) and with the examination of the conditions (Murray & Holmes 2014) that enable this voice to be raised and heard. From the first two chapters we learned that the "voice of medicine" can be a factor that encumbers the "voice of experience" to surface in (medical) encounters. But from the previous chapter we also learn that family as a significant horizon (or social structure) (Husserl 1965) for human living can complicate the sharing of the experience of suffering and the communication of need for help. Disease may threaten cherished ideas about falling in love and having a romantic relationship. It may menace expectations about how to be a good parent and a good partner or spouse. Families may hesitate to allow the voice of experience to become manifest because of the consequences (acceptance of change that affects the whole system) that may follow from taking that step.

The second point that we want to make refers to the definition of ethics of care as a moral theory that "implies that there is moral significance in the fundamental elements of relationships and dependencies in human life" (Sander-Staudt, 2011). The previous chapter suggests that there exists a gap between the 'place' where ethics of care as a moral theory starts (a positive acknowledgement of moral significance of relationships and dependencies) and the lived experiences of family life (relationships as sources of concern because relationships feel to be contested by illness). The families that we presented without exception grappled with allowing dependencies to become shared realities in the relational networks surrounding the person with MS. This might remind ethics of care of the fact that actual appraisal of the moral significance of relationships and dependencies might be preceded by a long process. In this process relational networks recreate themselves to make possible the emergence of a type of relationship that reflects the moral worth of being involved in an unequal relationship. Therefore, as a way of talking back to the ethics of care, we may emphasize the need to look at lived experience as a multidimensional space (metaphorically speaking) in which time lapse, imagination of one's position, the gaze of others are of utmost importance. Ethics of care that truly wants to be situational (Klaver, Elst & Baart 2013) should in other words not prematurely hail the merits of unequal relationships (Sander-Staudt, 2011). Instead it should carefully investigate the conditions that assure this type of relationships to emerges. With premature appraisal of the moral significance of dependency ethics of care might frustrate its own goal to promote the well-being of care-givers and care-receivers (Sander-Staudt 2011). In illness and care as lived phenomena the appreciation of dependency and suffering might be far less 'positive' than in care as a moral theory. A truly situational ethics of care takes this seriously and is ready to occupy a nuanced position on the moral significance of suffering and dependency.

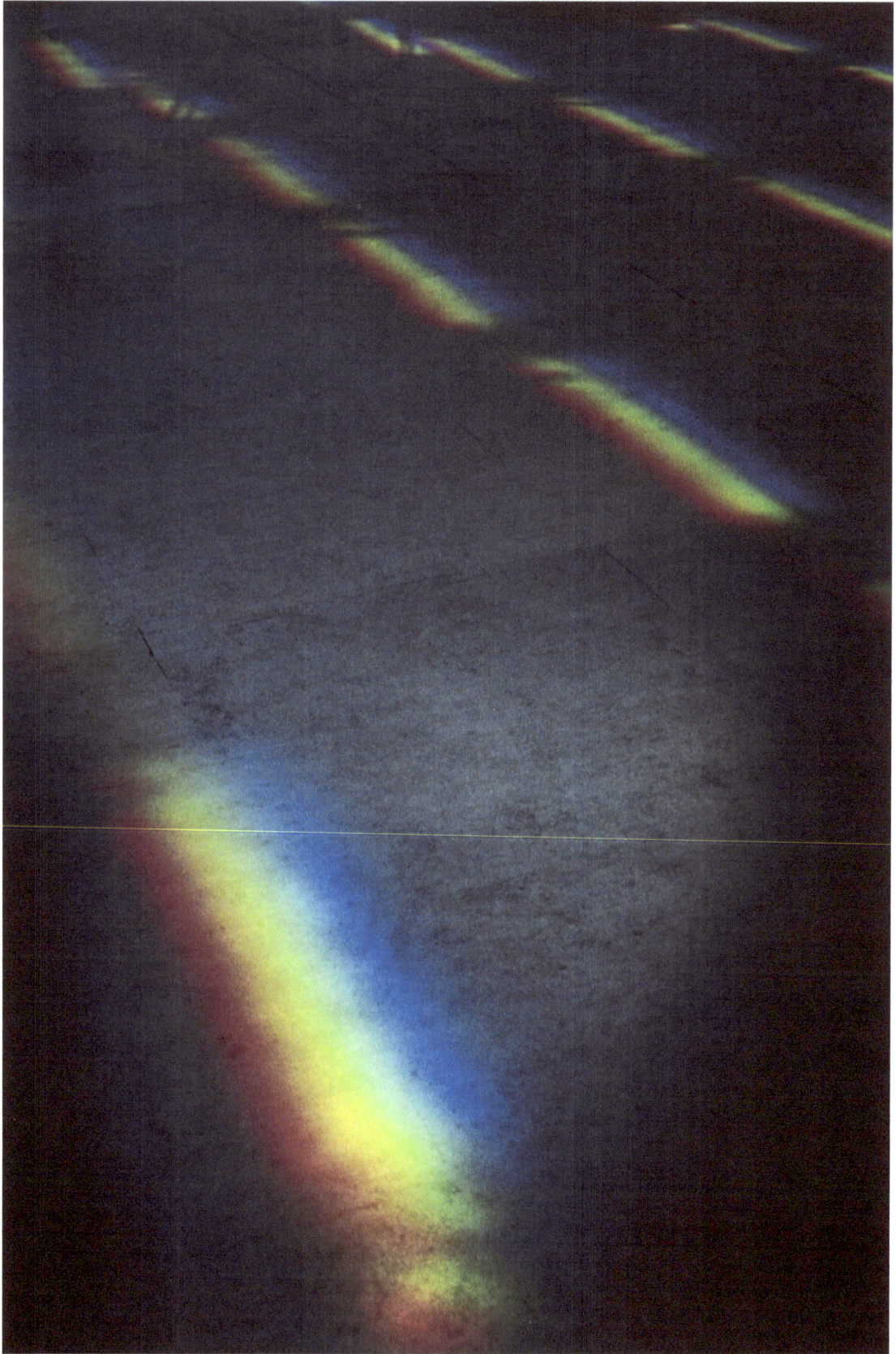

4. MS AND PAID WORK

Objective: This study explores the lived experience in their working lives of people with early stage multiple sclerosis (MS). Methods: Ten people at various stages in their careers (applying, employed, recently retired) who had been diagnosed with early stage MS were interviewed in open, in depth interviews. Transcriptions were analyzed following a phenomenological approach. Results: six themes were found: (1) the tiresome process of adjustment, (2) inventing ways to do your work, (3) feeling hurt about how others see your illness, (4) avoiding applying for jobs, (5) embracing retirement, and (6) mourning over lost work. Instead of relating these findings to mainstream theories that presuppose rather than investigate subjectivity (coping, self-management, skills), we generalize these findings by relating them to the psychodynamic model of work of Christophe Dejours. This model is a clinical theory that offers an account of the relations between subjectivity, work, and action. Conclusion: Current models of management and vocational rehabilitation maintain individual/group and body/mind dichotomies that don't exist in the lived experience of work and rehabilitation of people with MS. It is recommended that professionals offering supervision or vocational services to employees with early stage MS or other chronic conditions relativize these models while offering professional help, and that they revitalize the art of listening as an act of inclusion and acknowledgement.

Keywords: Qualitative Research, Perception, Relapsing-Remitting Multiple Sclerosis, Work, Employment

Ceuninck van Capelle, A. de, Visser, L. H., & Vosman, F. J. H. (2015) Multiple Sclerosis and Work: An Interpretative Phenomenological Analysis of the Perspective of Persons with Early Stage MS. Journal of Multiple Sclerosis (Foster City) 2:158. doi:10.4172/2376-0389.1000158

Introduction

A diagnosis of multiple sclerosis (MS), a chronic, incurable and sometimes progressive neurological illness (Compston & Coles, 2008) is usually an enormous shock for the person affected and for their intimate social circle. In time, the event might have far reaching consequences for their career and for their personal and public life (Pfleger et al., 2010a, 2010b). The medical, psychological, and social aspects of chronic illnesses have been studied widely, but scientific accounts of chronic illness written from the first person perspective remain rare. Most research in current medical and social sciences aims at the finding of quantifiable results, cause-effect relations, parameters and theories that predict the future. Within these types of studies, the subjectivity of the participant is exactly the phenomenon that needs to be ruled out. This state of affairs in the current practice of medical research however, doesn't rule out the possibility that the topic of subjectivity is not an important issue for the delivery of good care and hence of scientific exploration. We suggest that the growing interest in the last decades in comprehensive care and the patient perspective, rather indicates the opposite (Halper, 2008; Jason et al., 2014). Therefore, though we acknowledge the value of established methodologies, we think that the first-person perspective is a legitimate theme for scientific exploration and an appropriate object for the application of qualitative methods, which is indeed less common in medical sciences than their quantitative counterparts.

In the first person perspective, the patient diagnosed with the disease and involved in conversations about it describes what is happening to them and what is at stake following a diagnosis of MS. This is distinguished from the third person "helicopter" view of behavioral sciences such as psychology (Martin, 2011). Audulv's 'map' of recent qualitative research related to neurological illnesses (Audulv et al., 2014) and the systematic review of Sweetland on vocational rehabilitation for people with MS (Sweetland, Howse, & Playford, 2012) show that only a small part of recent studies on chronic neurological conditions is devoted to the exploration of the perspective of the person with the illness. Most research reflects other perspectives such as those of carers and of close relatives. In this paper we investigate how people with early stage MS experience their disease within their working lives.

MS impacts heavily on job retention. The participation in the labor market of people with MS is approximately half of that of the Dutch population in general (Kremer, Wevers, & Andries, 1997) and data for the United States show a similar situation (Julian, Vella, Vollmer, Hadjimichael, & Mohr, 2008). A few studies have explored the first person accounts of employed or recently unemployed persons with MS, for example Dyck (Dyck, 1995) who studied the patient's perspective by investigating the lives of two women with MS who had become recently unemployed. She focused on the complex intersection of body, place, space, gender and norms in their experience of home and neighborhood, and defined their world as one of shrinking places and silent spaces. Johnson et al. (Johnson et al., 2004) took a more generic approach to the patient's perspective by investigating the costs and the benefits of employment people with MS who were employed. Four themes emerged: (1) the cost-benefit economy of working, (2) fatigue and cognitive changes, (3) stress in the workplace, and (4) accommodations made to address barriers. Sweetland et al. (Sweetland, Riazi, Cano, & Playford, 2007) adopted a thematic approach by exploring in focus groups what people with MS require from a vocational rehabilitation service in terms of content and service delivery. They found two key issues: (1) managing performance and (2) managing expectations.

With our study we advance current research on MS and work, first by adopting the thematic focus of Sweetland (Sweetland et al., 2007) and Johnson (Johnson et al., 2004) but with a different approach. In their studies themes are arrived at by means of research questions about the needs, the costs and the benefits of employment. Even if the patients see these topics as relevant, they do not necessarily come close to capturing the full meaning of work for the MS patient. Therefore our approach is more open and does not initially demarcate specific points of interest. Rather, we aim to explore how the patients themselves prioritize issues. In this way we hope to find themes that are more representative of the perspective of people with MS and less the view of others such as policy makers and behavioral scientists. Secondly, our study adds to current research by adopting the lived experience approach of Dyck (Dyck, 1995) albeit with a different accent. Traditional investigations of lived experience use a more or less canonical 'grid' of elements that is used to investigate the collected data (Ashworth, 2006). In Dyck's study, the principal element investigated is space, while in older literature on the lived experience and MS, the body is an important element (Toombs, 1988). Similarly, our approach does not initially demarcate particular elements of the lived experience but rather aims at exploring how participants themselves prioritize these elements. By approaching the themes and the lived experience in this way, we approach phenomenology as an emancipatory methodology (Hodge, 2008) that aims to voice the experiences that matter most for people with illness. With this study we hope to gain deeper insight into how men and women with early stage MS experience and interpret their working life and career. This objective is concerned, in line with the qualitative design, with *meaning* and doesn't aim at, as is common in most medical studies, the testing of a hypothesis (Crouch & McKenzie, 2006; Mason, 2010). However, as a general assumption that undergirds this study, we hypothesize that colleagues, management, staff and social and health services view work differently than employees with MS, whose subjective, lived experience emerges from a complex set of social relations and everyday concerns, occurrences and situations.

Method

Design Our study began in 2012. We used purposeful sampling to include people with a definitive relapsing remitting MS diagnosis (McDonald et al., 2001) who had received their diagnosis a maximum of two years previously. Purposeful sampling differs from *random probability* sampling, the most current sampling method in medical and social sciences. Purposeful sampling is a form of *nonprobabilistic* sampling. It aims at the selection of information rich cases and the transferability of insight to other context, instead of statistical generalizability. In qualitative studies, nonprobabilistic sampling is common (Guest, Bunce, & Johnson, 2006; Patton, 2005). Recruitment was carried out by approaching patients from the records of a hospital's ambulatory MS care unit until we reached 10 participants. This number was in line with our aim of carrying out an explorative study and congruent with the demands of the chosen qualitative approach (Smith et al., 2009).

The validity, meaningfulness, and insights generated from qualitative enquiry have more to do with the information richness of the sample and the analytical capabilities of the researchers than with sample size (Patton, 2005). Yet, in qualitative studies in health care research, *theoretical saturation*, the point at which "no additional data are being found whereby the (researcher) can develop properties of the category" (Glaser & Strauss, 2009), has become the gold standard by which purposive sample sizes are determined (Guest et al., 2006; Mason, 2010; Tong, Sainsbury, & Craig, 2007). For phenomenological studies, samples consisting of a number of interviews in a range between 5 and 25 (Creswell, 1998) or 6 and 10 (Morse, 2000) are expected to lead to saturation. Guest et al. found in their dataset of sixty in-depth interviews with women in two West African countries that saturation occurred within the first twelve interviews, although basic elements for meta-themes were present as early as six interviews (Guest et al., 2006).

Data collection and Participants Three interviewers, the first and the third author and a resident neurologist[12], conducted conversational interviews in the homes of the participants. The interviews were conducted in Dutch, the native language of the participants and of the interviewers and the researchers. Following our open, explorative approach, we encouraged the participants to talk about what mattered most to them. The interviewers made use of a concise topic list that included work, personal situation, diagnosis and care. The participants were encouraged to prioritize topics, add them and discard them. The ethical committee of the St. Elisabeth Hospital in Tilburg approved the research and the patients gave informed consent for participation.

Data were gathered from 13 people: 10 people with MS and three partners that were asked by the person with MS to assist them with the interview. We granted this request, as is common in qualitative research on illness (Sakellariou et al., 2013). All participants resided in the Netherlands and the patients and the participating partners were Caucasian. The people with MS were aged 27-51 years. Two participants lived alone, eight lived with a spouse or a partner. Severity of symptoms, type of job and employment status varied. One was studying and applying for work, one had considered applying for a job but was actually retired, one was employed but on sick leave, one was employed but only working half of her contractual hours, two were employed without adjustments and three were retired. From the five employed participants, two received treatment with disease-modifying therapies. The remaining five participants who received treatment where unemployed at the time of the interview. Working experience varied from none at all up to several decades. Table 1 shows the profile of the participants. The table is arranged in ascending order of the participants' ages.

Table 1: Profile of the participants

Participant	Pseudonym	Interviewer	Gender	Age	Partner?	Career Stage	Profession
6	Kathy	1st author	F	27	yes	Studying,	musician

---

[12] See acknowledgements.

						applying	
3	Lucilia	DF	F	30	no	retired, considering applying	media designer
9	Shayne	1st author	F	31	yes	employed, on sick leave	cleaner
1	Livia	1st author	F	33	yes	employed, reduced hours	office worker
5	Lawrence	1st author	M	35	yes, Rosie[13]	retired	shoemaker
10	Renata	1st author	F	41	yes	employed	teacher
8	Savina	2nd author	F	43	yes	employed	secretary
7	Andrea	2nd author	F	45	yes	employed	librarian
2	Ricky	DF	M	46	Yes, Chandra[14]	retired	cleaner
4	Katherine	DF	F	51	Yes, Miljard[15]	retired	kitchen employee

Data analysis The analysis was guided by Interpretative Phenomenological Analysis (IPA), a qualitative approach (Smith et al., 2009). Data analysis consisted of three stages of inductive analysis of the digital audio files. In the first stage, shortly after each interview, the authors and a postdoctoral researcher[16] added, independently from each other, preparatory notes in Dutch in the right margins of the transcriptions. Within these notes, each researcher recorded free associations, pieces of theory, questions and possible related topics against specific excerpts of the transcription. Subsequently the transcriptions and notes were discussed in a plenary meeting. The cycle of interviewing, noting and discussing was repeated after each interview until the entire sample of 10 interviews was completed. In early 2013, a general meeting of the three

---

[13] Participating in the interview at the request of the participant.
[14] Participating in the interview at the request of the participant.
[15] Participating in the interview at the request of the participant.
[16] See acknowledgements.

authors at which emergent threads were identified concluded the first stage.

In 2013 and 2014 the first author entered the second stage by reworking the results of the first stage into a network of in vivo coded codes, supported by data analysis software Atlas.ti version 6.2, using a constant comparison method.

In the third stage that started in the autumn of 2014, guided by the network of codes and the methodological insights of IPA, the first author constructed six themes on career. Given the heterogeneity of career phases the participants appeared to be involved in, we analyzed the (from our phenomenological point of view) essential excerpts of the transcripts according to career stage as well as according to thematic kinship. This arrangement enabled us to include in the analysis, in a clear way, the divergent situational contexts of the participants while simultaneously allowing us to capture the significant nuances in similar themes across different career stages. The first author made a preliminary translation of the essential quotes falling under each theme. This translation was afterwards discussed and refined with the help of a professional translator (Van Nes et al., 2010).

Findings

Six themes were identified in the analysis: (1) the tiresome process of adjustment, (2) inventing ways to do your work, (3) feeling hurt about how others see your illness, (4) avoiding applying for jobs, (5) embracing retirement and (6) mourning over lost work. (Table 2) Each of these themes are described with quotes that illustrate the themes.

Table 2: Themes identified through analysis of interviews with 10 participants with early stage MS, ordered according to career stage and theme

Theme	Career stage at the time of the interview		
	Pre-Career	Mid-Career	Post-Career
The tiresome process of adjustment	Kathy	Shayne, Andrea	Katherine, Lawrence
Inventing ways to do your work		Livia, Savina	
Feeling hurt about how others see your illness	Lucilia, Kathy	Andrea	Lawrence
Avoiding job application	Lucilia	Andrea	

Embracing retirement			Lawrence
Mourning over lost work			Katherine, Ricky

The tiresome process of adjustment. The onset of MS meant for the participants the start of a period of making adjustments in the domain of work and income. Kathy had just finished her music exams with excellent grades then she fell ill and also 'fell' into a social benefit. From there she received coaching from the social services to get a job at places she felt very uneasy with. Kathy commented:

"Well, they do a lot to get you a job, but the places where they put you don't really make you happy." [6:84] "At the end, when I was at the point of escaping from benefits, the woman, a job coach, said to me: 'I really hope you find something else, because this doesn't fit you at all'. That workplace was a factory." {6:85}[17]

Shayne, a cleaner, already had a longstanding relationship with her employer when she fell ill. As with Kathy the course of adjustment was not smooth. A first attempt to adjust failed:

"About the UWV[18], I have not a single good word to say. If you need something, I don't care what, it's a worthless institute. (…) The UWV closed [at one point] my case and left my boss – I have known my boss for a long time, he knows my situation – to cope alone with all the legal stuff, rehabilitation, sick leave, etc. [He was unable to manage all of this] so I just continued my cleaning work." {9:91}

After some months however, Shayne had an intensive meeting with the doctor in which she realized that she had ignored her illness for too long:

"At that moment I chose for myself. So I said, 'sorry boss, this doesn't work for me anymore. It's me first now, because otherwise I just can't carry on.'" {9:94}

Andrea, a librarian, also told her manager that she couldn't carry on as she had done. Changing her working circumstances appeared, however, to be a demoralising affair:

"After a lot of hassle I managed to get a dispensation from that work [that entailed standing] for one hour at noon while I did sedentary work instead. This was an adaptation that was added to my contract and to my personnel file…. I managed to get agreement for this arrangement with the support of my occupational physician (…). In the recent past I

---

[17] {transcription : quotation}
[18] *Uitvoeringsinstituut Werknemers Verzekeringen*, Dutch Social Insurance Institute.

had been awarded a bonus a couple of times: 'You are a good employee and we are happy with you', but when a thing like this happens to you, you fall ill, nobody can do anything about it, and they are unresponsive. That frustrates me enormously. {7:97}.

Katherine, working as a dishwasher in the kitchen of a care institution, also had a troubled relationship with her line manager in trying to get her work adapted to suit her new circumstances:

"They don't understand me, or they don't want to understand me, or they don't understand MS. And that relationship didn't go very well. (…)' And after only six months, he said, 'When things are not going well with you, your diplomas fit you for nothing other than functioning as domestic help.' And I said: 'That's not for me, I'm not able to do that.'" {4:21}

Inventing ways to do your work. Livia, Andrea and Savina were working at the time of the interview. Livia, an office worker at a major manufacturing company, and Savina, a secretary in the local town hall, told how they dealt with MS on an average working day:

Livia: "I have a contract [to work] 40 hours, but actually I manage only 20 hours, so I do the same work in half the time. (…) I found a way to [organise my] work. When people have a question for me – questions by email are the easiest to handle – and I don't see any urgency, I don't respond, unless they get back to me [another time and I know] that it is important for them. This economises [on my work] quite a lot [laughter]. So this is how I can do my [40 hour] job in 20 hours. {1:58}.

But besides her own 'tricks', Livia found that the help of others was very important too for holding on to her job:

"You notice the small things. Somebody at the office came to me and said: 'I asked you to draft that article, but, you know, I will just do it myself'. [Or] when I was assigned to a meeting, [I liked the fact that someone said to me], 'you know, I'll take that.'" {1:58}

For Savina, personal perseverance was needed to get up and go out to work in spite of her illness:

"Sometimes I wake up and think: 'I'm so tired', but then I boost myself up, and I manage to do it." {8:133}

Feeling hurt about how others see your illness. Four participants said how they felt hurt about the way in which others saw their illness. Lucilia, a media designer and photographer, dreamed of starting her own business. After her graduation, however, she was assigned to a rehabilitation project because her complaint prevented her from entering the labor market.

"But they kicked me out [of the project], I was really devastated. [They said:] … 'Well, you're sick. So you can't …. Goodbye!' They really made a mistake." {3:182} "It was a really bad blow [for me]" {3:273}

For Kathy a blow came quite unexpectedly from a friend and colleague after a failed application at a renowned orchestra. Kathy told how her friend commented on the outcome of her application:

"'You know, Kathy, perhaps it's just better that things have turned out like this, because if you had been hired, you would not have persevered because you have MS. One doesn't even stand a chance with the medical tests with asthma, let alone in your position!' Well, then I was really angry! Usually I never tell people my opinions directly, but on this occasion I told her the truth. I felt really embarrassed." {6:60}

Andrea related how she felt awkward and sad when she heard how a colleague had commented on her illness:

"At the outset a colleague said to me: 'When I see you, I only see MS.' I replied: 'I really regret that. Of course, it belongs to me and it will never leave me. But I hope I'm more than that.'" {7:85}

For Lawrence, who used to be an orthopedic shoemaker, he was alienated by the attitude towards his illness of someone at the UWV office:

"I received an invitation from the UWV to get a work capacity interview. They immediately asked me for my plans. I replied: 'Something secretarial'. And then they said: 'Grab that pen and strike that particular entry field. You will never be able to work again.' That was a strange idea to me because I had never experienced such a weird thing before, that someone would say to me: 'you will never resume work again.' And they also asked me: 'Who do you expect to hire you?'" {5:32}

Avoiding applying for jobs. Two participants told how they felt MS inhibited them from entering the labor market (Lucilia) or to make a career move (Andrea). Lucilia:

"I was very glad when the people from the UWV said to me: 'So you want your own business? Well, try it!' But recently I had to take a step backwards." {3:197} "I am stressed, not able to function properly, and very much affected by disabling fatigue. (...) very annoying. So I decided to apply for a job first and try [to start my own business] again in two years?" {3:189}.

But at the time of the interview, Lucilia was still not applying for jobs:

"Yes, but making that step ... setting up challenges I probably can't meet...what if I'm at the office and I'm hit by disabling fatigue? These are all new things I will have to address, so I am thinking of myself a bit: may I not have some extra time staying at home?" {3:264}

Similarly, Andrea said:

"At one particular moment there was a teaching vacancy at the ROC[19], and I fancied applying, but I didn't dare , because of my MS. I was supposed to study and to teach, new things. Yes, I think, it [MS] inhibits me from taking such a step." {7:100}. "And family life is pretty busy here, so I don't think making such a move is a good idea." {7:102}

Embracing retirement. Lawrence and his wife Rosie told how they had reflected on the costs and benefits of being employed and how they had decided to apply for a social benefit:

"And yes, on one hand I had some motivation to work. But on the other, considering the economic situation and the response [of employers] when I applied [during my reintegration trajectory], I thought: 'well, let's strike that entry field because then, in any case, I'll know what I'm doing'". {5:47}

Mourning over lost work. For Katherine and Ricky, the onset of MS meant the end of several decades of working as a breadwinner. They therefore missed their work a lot. Katherine:

"After the rehabilitation center's assessment, having consulted the occupational physician and the psychologist, I decided to make early application for a full WIA[20] benefit, because, given the findings of the assessment, there would not be work for me anyway: not being able to work in a team, not being able to listen to music, having a maximum

---

[19] *Regionaal Opleidingscentrum*, Regional Education Centre.
[20] *Werk en Inkomen naar Arbeidsvermogen*, Act on Work and Income According to Work Capacity.

concentration span of half an hour, the sum of all that … So the occupational physician said: 'Lets apply.' And that guy from Human Resources said: 'Well, okay, we will fix the paperwork.' And off he went. (…) After 15 years of loyal service. My work meant everything for me." {4:35}

Ricky's wife Chandra related:

"They checked [his abilities to work], his eyes, but he can't see very well, he can't concentrate, and he can't deal with busy places, so many things. Finding a job [while having so many limitations] is actually impossible." {2:28}

Ricky added:

"It was really difficult for me to cope with that. Let's see, I'm 46 now, I started to work when I was 12 years old, and worked right up until that day, and then – nothing. Every day I went to work at seven in the morning, was busy until, say, eight or nine at night. And now – nothing. That's tough, isn't it?" {2:34}

Discussion

Summarizing the results of analysis To answer the research question about how people live with early stage MS, we interviewed 10 patients, diagnosed no more than two years prior to the interview. In our sample we found that early MS wasn't associated with one specific career stage but affected people at the beginning of their career, in its midst, or else truncated their career with early retirement. Participants at all three career stages had experienced hurtful situations in relation to how others understood their illness and interpreted their return to work, either supervised by the UWV or by their employer, as a tiresome process. Participants in pre- as well as mid-career stages worried about the consequences of their illness for their career in the future. Evaluating the course of their already-terminated careers, one participant saw the stability associated with living on incapacity for work benefits as an advantage , while for two others, missing their work was the dominant perspective.

What should be the aim of qualitative analysis of the first-person perspective? Qualitative research on the first-person perspective is meant to excavate the themes, patterns, understandings and insights that characterize this perspective. In IPA this excavation takes the form of the investigation of lived experiences, including their particularities and the specific contexts in which they occur. Like other methods, IPA aims at establishing generalizations but, according to Smith et al., it "prescribes a different way of establishing those generalizations. It locates them in the particular and hence develops them more cautiously" (Smith et al., 2009). However, despite this exhortation to proceed slowly and with caution, recently Murray and Holmes (Murray & Holmes, 2014) argued that most applications of IPA actually offer straightforward descriptions of lived experiences, without "taking account of subject formation and of the context within which the subject might appear as the bearer of an ethical claim". Within the small body of qualitative research pertaining to illness and work, a similar point is made by Tiedtke et al. (Tiedtke, Rijk, Donceel, Christiaens, & Casterlé, 2012) and also Van Hal et al. (Van Hal, Meershoek, Rijk, & Nijhuis, 2012) on behaviorism in models of return to work (De Rijk, Janssen, Van Lierop, Alexanderson, & Nijhuis, 2009; Franche & Krause, 2002; Krause & Ragland, 1994; Prochaska, DiClemente, & Norcross, 1992), and the emphasis on skills in vocational interventions for the unemployed (Audhoe, Hoving, Sluiter, & Frings-Dresen, 2010). They maintain, each in their own way, that much research focusses on self-management (Detaille, Gulden, Engels, Heerkens, & Dijk, 2010; Lorig & Holman, 2003; Minis et al., 2014; Munir, Leka, & Griffiths, 2005; Schulman-Green et al., 2012), coping (Johnson et al., 2004), needs (Sweetland et al., 2007) and skills and generally overlooks the subject that makes skills, processes and behaviors actually 'happen'. This subject however is much more unstable, much more subject to doubt, affection, and interpretation than is generally accounted for. We agree with this position and hold that qualitative analysis of the first-person perspective should focus more on the process of subject formation itself.

Understanding MS and work as central for subjectivity: The psychodynamic model of Dejours
Aligning with a concern for subjectivity, we think that Dejours' psychodynamic model of work (Dejours & Deranty, 2010), a clinical approach that focusses on the dynamic relationship between subjectivity, work, and action, offers a reliable route to generalizing the findings of our data without losing sight of the theme of subject formation. Building on the works of psychoanalyst Le Guillant (Le Guillant, 1984) and ergonomist Wisner (Wisner, 1972; Wisner, Veil, & Dejours, 1985), in the last decades Dejours has developed a model that identifies four ways in which work is central for the formation of subjectivity: (1) the centrality of work in

relation to the subject's mental health, (2) the centrality of work in the structure of relationships between men and women, (3) the centrality of work in relation to the community, and (4) the centrality of work in relation to the theory of knowledge. We think two parts of this model (part 1 and 3) apply to the results of our analysis.

The first aspect of the work – subjectivity relationship consists in uncovering the specific conditions that turn the relationship with work into one of sadness or joy. The influence of work on one's individual experience plays out on an individual as well as a social level. At the individual level the subject experiences the resistance of the world (including the physical aspect as well its complexity) when she or he tries to accomplish the assigned tasks. Solving the difficulties and accomplishing the tasks leads not only to appropriation of the world but also of the body and of the self. On the social level, Dejours points to the importance of one's peers recognizing one's achievements as an essential part in the development of identity. Our findings relate to the individual level in this respect that the temporary but frequent waves of fatigue made the participants doubt the extent to which they were actually able, or would be able in the future, to accomplish the assigned tasks. Concerning the social level, one participant (Livia) felt proud that, with the help of her peers, she had managed to adapt her work to the constraints of her illness. The importance of recognition was also felt by other participants, but predominantly in a negative way. It was felt that stigmatizing attitudes towards illness blocked colleagues or managers from seeing (and recognizing) the actual efforts that were made and what was accomplished (social level). Being deprived of work was seen by two participants (Ricky and Katherine) as a great personal loss, hence confirming the centrality of work for subjectivity.

The second aspect of the work – subjectivity and relationships (third element in the model of De-jours) – points to the fact that work is not only about getting things done but also about cooperation with others. Work, according to Dejours, is "not only production, it is also learning to live together". Work requires a minimum of consideration of others and of conviviality. However, with one poignant exception (Livia), the perspective on work as a social activity seems to be remarkably absent in our sample. Dejours says, however, that the social aspect of work ("effective forms of *cooperation* that should be differentiated from prescribed forms of *coordination*[21]") is obscured and damaged by the currently dominant systemic or functionalist approaches of work organization. These latter approaches seem to have been experienced in

---

[21] Our emphasis.

great measure by the participants. Some of them felt their treatment by UWV was depersonalized, they were just numbers to UWV; others lamented the bureaucratic or formalistic angles taken by their employers. Generally (with the exception of Livia), the participants felt that their situation was more viewed as an individual and functionalistic problem than as an issue of cooperation and conviviality.

Implications of this study for vocational professionals Vocational professionals work for the most part with medical, psychological and organizational models that just presuppose the subject and understand body, self, and world as relatively static, objective and pre-given entities. This study, however, like some previous ones (Dyck & Jongbloed, 2000; Dyck, 1995; Finlay, 2003), points to the contrary. Identity, body, and world are dynamic and interrelated.

It is therefore recommended that professionals primarily concerned with the body, for example vocational physicians, relativize the current emphasis on the functionalist aspect of the body. This emphasis even finds expression in Dutch social law as a quantified notion of an individual's remaining capacity for work. But as inability to perform specific tasks at work emerges, it isn't just a matter of applying the law or of compensating for loss of income. The emerging situation has a profound effect on identity and relationships with the world. From a phenomenological point of view the importance of remaining connected with the world through physical activity can therefore be seen to be paramount. It should, however, not be confounded with the functionalist argument that work serves well-being or with the "logic of activation" (Vossen & Gestel, 2015). Demotion, civic voluntarism and regular daytime activities might be useful instruments for continued activity and are preferable to the lack of activity that often goes alongside living on social benefits.

Likewise, it is recommended that professionals primarily concerned with psychological and motivational issues relativize the current mentalism that runs through popular approaches such as empowerment (Varekamp et al., 2009), by acknowledging the intertwining of mental phenomena with the body and the environment (Dyck, 1995; Murray & Holmes, 2014). Finally, it is recommended that professionals with managerial responsibilities relativize the current exaltation of individual performance and acknowledge the role of co-operation and conviviality in the workplace. Organizational aspects may very well contribute to the alleviation as well as to the aggravation of the effect of MS on work. We suggest here the importance of the "art of listening", previously identified by Van Hal et al. (Van Hal et al., 2012) and Dejours and Garnet (Dejours & Gernet, 2012) as a preferred device or instrument for inclusion and acknowledgement.

Limitations of this study and suggestions for future research In research on occupational rehabilitation, concepts that presuppose rather than research subjectivity (skills, needs, coping, empowerment, self-management, etc.) display an overwhelming presence. Studies that conceptualize subjectivity and identity as dynamic, contextual, and interpretational issues are few and far between, and those that exist seem to focus principally on establishing that subjectivity is currently neglected in the research. Establishing this point is a main concern also for our study too and this is a strength as well as a limitation. In order to advance research of the first-person perspective – critical (including our own) as well as mainstream approaches - it might be necessary to (1) incite a broader awareness in first-person research for the current lack of attention for the formation of the subject, to (2) reorganize the currently scattered (but actually affiliated) research on contextual subjectivity across diverse life domains (health, work, intimate life, etc.) into a more unified framework for research on subjectivity and to (3) bridge the divide between 'mainstream' and 'critical' research by investigating how broadly accepted concepts like "coping" and "empowerment" relate to the subtleties and particularities of subject formation. A necessary progression of this study is to investigate more thoroughly the relationship between subjectivity, work, and action, specifically for MS. Dejours' psychodynamic model of work offers a generic account and doesn't address the particular the situation of workers with a disease, let alone of workers with MS. Although we think, as we mentioned above , that Dejours' model offers a convincing path for the generalization of the findings of our data, this study doesn't, conversely, answer the question what configuration of subjectivity, work, and action is characteristic for employees with MS. Future, comparative, research on workers with neurological and other diseases is needed to discover the defining characteristics of the 'fingerprint' with which MS marks the professional life of persons living with this disease. We expect that MS-related episodic disability in combination with fear about the future development of the disease course might be found among the identifying elements. This remains, however, to be investigated.

Finally, our study applies a single interview per participant design (Morse, 2000). The participants, however, presented their experiences without exception as a process or a succession of events. This finding suggests that for future research on MS and work, a longitudinal design, with multiple interviews conducted over a period of months or even years, is recommendable and could offer more detailed and sustained insights in the (development of the) meaning of work for people with MS. A particularly interesting focus for a longitudinal design of would be the presence or absence of the topic of treatment with disease-modifying therapies within the experience of work. Physicians greatly value adherence to treatment and there is evidence that, notwithstanding the complex relations between MS and work, receiving treatment supports job retention and reduces the duration of sick leaves and utilization of medical care (Lage, Castelli-Haley, & Oleen-Burkey, 2005; Rajagopalan, Brook, Beren, & Kleinman, 2010; Ziemssen, Hoffman, Apfel, & Kern, 2008). However, how do employees with MS understand the relation between disease-modifying therapies and work? Do they have the same views like their doctors or do they disagree? Since we didn't control our sample for treatment with disease-modifying therapies, future (longitudinal) studies should address this gap.

Conclusion Our phenomenological analysis of interviews with 10 people with early stage MS has yielded six themes: (1) the tiresome process of adjustment, (2) inventing ways to do your work, (3) feeling hurt about how others see your illness, (4) avoiding applying for jobs, (5) embracing retirement, and (6) mourning over lost work. Unsatisfied with regular conceptual approaches to illness and work that presuppose rather than investigate subjectivity, we turned to the psychodynamic model of work of Dejours to generalize our findings without losing the particularities of contexts in which subjectivity takes form. Two elements of this model, the centrality of work in relation to the subject's mental health and the centrality of work in relation to the community, emerged as applicable to the generalization of the results of our analysis. It is recommended that professionals offering leadership or vocational services to people with early MS and other chronic conditions relativize the current functionalist and individualist approaches to work and acknowledge the relevance of conviviality, cooperation, and of the actual intertwining of self, body and world in the work environment.

"My work meant everything for me."

> In a second interview with my line manager the Human Resources manager was also present. And then that guy from the Human Resources department said to me:
> 'And now I want you to say for yourself what's the matter with you.'
> and I said:
> 'No I'm just not able to do that.'
> And then my [also present] husband assisted me [and said]:
> 'She can't … say it.'
> [Interviewer asks] 'Were you [husband] there too?
> [Husband]: 'Yes'
>
> [Participant #4 resumes]: And then the [also present at the exit interview] occupational physician said:
> 'Well, let's …'
>
> - And I had discussed this point previously with him and the psychologist, I decided to make an early application for a full WIA benefit, because, given the findings of the assessment [of capacity for work], there would not be work for me anyway: not being able to work in a team, not being able to listen to music, having a maximum concentration span of half an hour, the sum of all that …-
>
> So the occupational physician said:
>
> 'Lets apply.'
>
> And that guy from Human Resources said:
> 'Well, okay, we will fix the paperwork.'
> And off he went. After 15 years of loyal service. My work meant everything to me." [P4:28-35]

In the previous chapters we studied how people with MS experience illness and care in the contexts of professional care and of families. In the fourth chapter we turned to a third context – professional life – in which illness and care appear as phenomena of the patient experience of MS. As an analogue to our approach to care and families as relational networks we understand professional life as a social phenomenon (Dejours 2010) wherein people can but not necessarily do appear to each other as real persons. We would like to use the final excursus de in this study to outline how a strategic handling of regulations for sick leave and early retirement by both employers and people with MS may also provide another barrier for the voice of experience to emerge. The previously, in the introduction, introduced distinction between spoken language as a means to an end and as a phenomenon that unfolds in a relational scene of address from our adapted version of IPA (Murray & Holmes 2015, Holmes 2015) can be used to clarify how this happens.

How language can be used as a tool and as a means to an end is clearly visible. Participant #4 (Katherine) had prepared the exit interview carefully with her psychologist and her occupational physician. A pivotal role in this preliminary meeting was assigned to a (medical and psychological) report about Katherine's capacity for work. Judging from this report Katherine decides to head in the interview with her managers towards an early application for a full WIA benefit. Far from a "relational scene of address" (Murray & Holmes 2014) the interview is rather a strategic game in which Katherine and her allies use spoken language (aligned according to the written assessment of capacity for work) as a tool to get what she wants. Since Katherine feels her capacity to phrase her thoughts to be diminished her husband and the occupational physician help her. The use of language remains however invariantly instrumental, but at the end of Katherine's account of her exit interview the participant changes her tone of voice: "And off he went. After 15 years of loyal service. My work meant everything to me." This sentence isn't meant to achieve a goal but rather expresses the pain and the loss that losing work for Katherine entails. But the phrase is not uttered during the exit interview but during the research interview. That interview hence functions here more likely as a *patch* to cover the (by necessity) missing moral aspect (losing work as a personal loss) of the exit interview (because of the preferred instrumental approach). It serves as more than only an intersubjective *correlate* for the event that was originally experienced as individual (Murray & Holmes 2014).

We learn from the final chapter of this study that besides the distinction between the "biomedical voice" and "the voice of experience" (Toombs 1988, Frank 2000) in language as a phenomenon also a parallel distinction between instrumental and relational types in spoken language as a phenomenon applies. The emotional and financial stakes in professional environments that are affected by disease are always high. This may encourage persons with MS and other participants of (professional) networks to prefer an instrumental approach to contact (that allows you to get want you want) over an expressive approach (that allows others to see who you are). In each of the three situations that we have explored in this study – professional care, the family, and occupation – the tension between instrumental and expressive applications of language by patient and others alike is noticeable. Physicians try to pair the correct transmission of objective medical information with a mentality that seeks to understand medical care as a human response to a call from a fellow person for help. Patients need the insights of medicine to soften the effects of disease but also struggle to find meaning in illness and care for their own lives. Finally, the tension between instrumental and expressive applications of language arises in situations wherein persons with MS have to decide about the preservation of positions in families and work

94

circles. The costs of becoming expressive and relational about illness and need for care might be substantial. But also staying within the borders of sedimented language and conventions comes with a price. A gap between experienced identity and the taking of a position that hides it (and hence confirms the *status quo*) may trouble daily life with disease as much as the disruption of relational network that may follow the *coming out* as a person with MS. However the burden of disease is in the first instance taken by the patient alone while in the second it is the *network* that takes it. Within the context of the idea that communities should be stages at which people can appear to each other as real persons (Klaver, Van Elst & Baart 2013) the second way of dealing with MS – as a community rather than as an individual – is preferable.

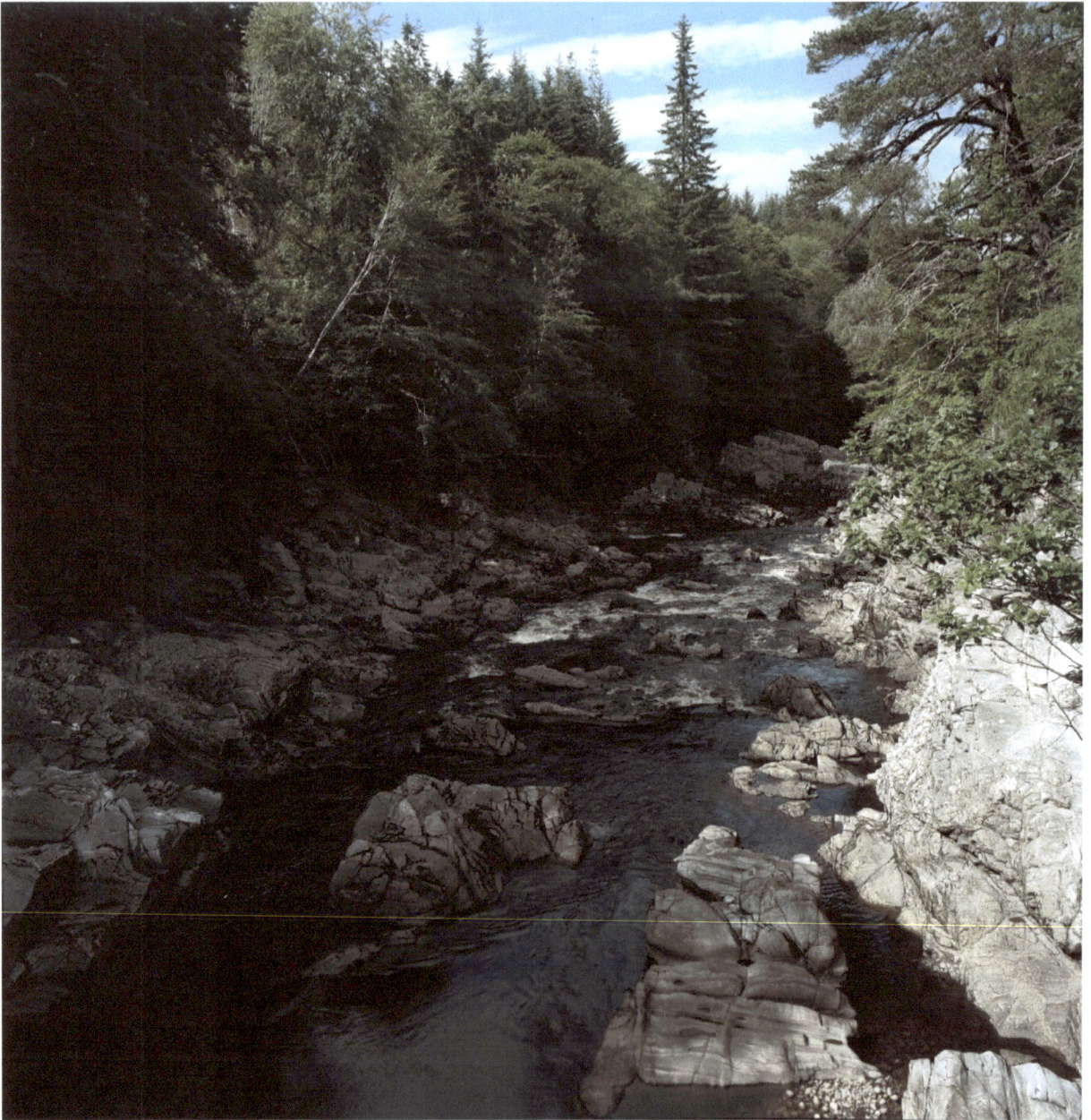

DISCUSSION

The concluding section of this study opens with a summary of the methods and the findings of this study. Next we reflect on the question how ethics of care can work as an approach for the improvement of health care. Following a comparison with "patient centred care" as a drive for change we suggest that ethics of care contributes to good care by extending the analytical lens. We display an example of how this works by presenting the main insights from the four chapters of this study as ingredients for an understanding of physicians and patients that is more differentiated and more realistic than other approaches (paternalistic and progressive). We continue with an evaluation of some recent objections that Sholl and Gergel raised against phenomenology as a method to clarify issues in medicine. After we have clarified our positions toward these objections we reflect on the contribution of our phenomenological ethics of care to the way ethics of care understand the moral significance of relationships. This contribution lies in the insight that the lived moral significance of relationships seems to have varied degrees of intensity. We conclude with recommendations for professional and informal care for people with recently-diagnosed MS.

Summary of the method and the findings of this study

Our phenomenological analysis of lived experiences of persons with early stage MS (Smith et al. 2009) started with the design of the research interview as a relational scene of address that functioned as the intersubjective correlate for the events that where originally experienced by the participant as an individual (Murray & Holmes 2014). Already begun during the interview was a process of contextualization, apprehending and clarifying of lived experiences (Bevan, 2014). This was continued by the analysis team and culminated in the four research articles that constitute the backbone of this study. Depending on the nature of the fragment of the interview (as represented in audio recording and transcription) we applied a small collection of additional concepts to deepen and enhance the threefold process of phenomenological reduction. This collection included the distinction between "the biomedical voice" and "the voice of experience" (Toombs 1988), the ideas of lived body, time and place (Toombs 1988), the distinction between instrumental and expressive usage of spoken language (Murray & Holmes, 2013, 2014) and the idea of relationships as horizons for human experience (Husserl 1965).

The findings of this study involve descriptions of illness and care as lived by persons with MS in the environments of professional care, families and professional life. These environments are approached in this study as subjective accounts of relational lifeworlds. We consider these descriptions and interpretations to account for "the voice of experience" previously defined as the voice that communicates suffering and that tells what is happening in terms of impact on this particular person and those with whom they are most intimately involved.

During the process of diagnosis, the world of the person with MS becomes a contested place. The body feels different and doesn't move like it used to do, which hampers self-confidence and self-reliance. The places where the patient is brought to are unknown and full of potential threats. Regarding DMT the participants struggle to take a personal stance when faced with complex statistical information on medical benefits and risks. Some feel scared about administering injections. In a few participants that had accepted treatment fear of injections and doubts about efficacy continued to resurface. But most of the participants that had accepted DMT managed to make it part of their ordinary lives.

Relationships. Most participants took pride in caring for others (children, partner, parents) and where in charge of their households at the time that MS started to affect their family lives. Fatigue and cognitive problems are felt to interfere severely with their ability to care for others. Some participants outline "help" as a theme of its own. Accepting help from mother or partner means for them that their illness and limitations to become more real. Some participants highlight awkward attitudes (including well-meant 'offers' to help) to their illness, overstating their position as a patient, misapprehending symptoms and airing ignorance about MS without even knowing it. MS feels for four participants to spoil emotional intimacy between them and their children or mother. The lost harmony in the family is experienced in feelings of distance and isolation. Moreover, as far as the participants had been able to see what was on their family members' mind, it offered little encouragement. Sad family members, in the eyes of the participants, often struggled with feelings of fear grief, and confusion to which they had no more an answer than the participants themselves.

Professional life. Regarding professional life we found that early MS is not associated with one specific career stage but affects people at the beginning of their career, in the midst of it, or else truncates their career with early retirement. Participant's at all three career stages experience hurtful situations in relation to how others understand their illness and interpreted their return to work, either supervised by the UWV or by their employer, as a tiresome process. Participants in pre- as well as mid-career stages worry about the consequences of their illness for their career in the future. Evaluating the course of their already-terminated careers, one participant sees the stability associated with living on incapacity for work benefits as an advantage, while for two others, missing their work is the dominant perspective.

Improving care by extending the analytical lens

This study is – being a part of the MLZ program (Baart, Vosman et al. 2015) – meant to make a contribution to the transformation and improvement of hospital-based care. The theoretical framework of this program was ethics of care and these ethics constituted the theoretical background to this study. We underline at this point that the focus of this background differs substantially from the focus of "patient centered care" (Gerteis, 1993; Institute of Medicine, 2001) that is at the moment the drive behind many programs for improvement of care around the world (Eijk et al., 2011). The global idea of "patient centered care" is a shift from paternalistic care towards patient centered care. In paternalistic care the physician is in the lead and the patient is a silent receiver of care. Although this idea still holds for critical care, during the 1990s the idea emerged that for most forms of care a shift towards the patient as the new center of medicine was appropriate. Ethics of care as a concept for improvement of care implies a shift but this shift is not from one stakeholder (the physician) to the other (the patient) but rather aims towards a form of care that transcends any approach to care in terms of (antagonistic) groups. The *relationship* between providers and receivers of care is the factor considered to be critical for the development of good care. The reason behind this is that caring, i.e. the practice of caring, is seen as relational – good care emerging from within that relationship (Van Heijst 2011). However one could however legitimately ask what could be the substance of this critical factor. We think that one way to understand this substance is to see the focus on relationships as a method to improve our vision of care. Ethics of care can in other words be used as a tool to extent the analytical lens (Philip, 2013). We will elaborate now on this claim by showing how our view gets broadened when we take the patients' experiences seriously.

The chapters of this study were interlaced with four excursuses that presented each a longer fragment from the audio transcriptions that was meant to magnify the main insights from the preceding chapter. Now we use three of these excursuses to display how emphasis on professional care, families, and professional life *as relational networks lived by patients* indeed enhances current visions on care. We begin by turning to conceptualizations of the patient. Sometimes is the patient is still conceived of as the silent and passive receiver of care. This was also the state affairs in the fragment in the first excursus. The classification of her appeal for care as an emergency case overwhelmed P9 (Shayne) as did the pace of the sequence of events that followed. But even though the P9 readily followed the recommendations of her health care providers it became clear that the concept of "adherence" only tells half the story. The presence of an underlying but audible "voice of experience" was evident in the fragment and also in the other interviews. In the fragment about the process of hospitalization this voice surfaced in the request to delay hospitalization for a few hours to get ready. In consumerist approaches, besides "adherence", another common approach to the agency of the patient, the patient is not a passive receiver but rather imagined as the active promotor of his or her health. But the second excursus showed that concepts like "preference" and "satisfaction" (these concepts are often linked with consumerist approaches) account again for no more than part of the story. P10 (Renata) didn't shop to get the best product but rather searched for care that matched with her person and the story of her life. Finally also the fourth excursus indicates an extension of the understanding of the patient by showing that besides providers of care patients too may opt for a more practical track trough the care system.

Physicians in relationships. Emphasis on professional care, families, and professional life as relational networks lived by patients has also differentiated the picture of the physician. The exploration of the evaluation of providers of care by receivers of care is relatively new and this is even more so for an exploration of this evaluation using qualitative methods (rankings and ratings being currently the most common methods for evaluation). The first two excursuses showed a picture of a doctor that was not only valued because of his learning in the technical and medical details in current MS medicine (the usual basis for evaluating who is a good doctor). He was also valued because of his ability to combine this learning with sensitivity for the specific needs and concerns of the patient in front of him. In the appendix to this study, Van Iersel (2016) beautifully expands on this point. We must admit, however, that the fourth excursus contains a problem. P4 (Katherine) values her occupational physician not because he is skilled *and* sensitive. She rather considers him to be a good doctor *by virtue of* being skilled (in guiding her through the maze of the social care system to achieve early retirement). We hit here at a fundamental divide in thinking about medicine as a human art and as a natural science. Can medicine be accomplished as a moral endeavor by natural science alone or is it indeed in want of human sciences (like phenomenology) to achieve that? Or is phenomenology not the approach to bring the two together?

Answering recent objections against phenomenology as a key to understanding medicine

Recently Gergel (2012) and Sholl (2015) have argued that Toombs, Zaner, Carel and other phenomenologists overestimate the role of phenomenology for the practice of medicine as a human art. Without denying that the discipline that was founded by Husserl has some merit for contemporary medicine, they maintain that many contributions of phenomenology to medicine (as a moral approach to care and as a qualitative method) are flawed. Gergel (2012) motivates this claim by contrasting four claims of phenomenology regarding medicine that are subsequently downplayed or relativized. These insights are (1) phenomenology can help us to understand illness and the individual themselves (2) through attaching primary importance to the direct experiencing of phenomena we suspend pre-existing assumptions and gain fresh understanding of illness (*epochè*), (3) a phenomenological approach to illness can lessen or prevent the way in which illness and medical treatment compromise the integrity of the individual's sense of self, and (4) phenomenology is radically different from other medical approaches. Sholl (2015) extends Gergel's critique by complementing her evaluation with two additional points: (a) a critique of how phenomenologists (mis)represent the viewpoints of their adversaries (naturalists) and (b) a questioning of the concept of "normality" in phenomenological accounts of health and illness.

Above we raised the question if medicine can be accomplished as a moral endeavor by natural science alone or rather needs complementation by human sciences (like phenomenology) to achieve that. The answer of Gergel and Sholl would be that natural science can almost completely account for a humane (which means for them an individualized and contextualized) medicine. For Gergel phenomenology has indeed its place but should be conceived of rather as a "philosophical arena for considering questions of how to integrate the context and values of individual perspectives into general conceptions of illness and treatment". Phenomenology should hence stop its "sectarian polemic" against evidence-based medicine. Sholl sparingly adds to this that phenomenology can "provide some useful insights into what it is like to experience health and illness, insights which might be able to benefit from the trained analytic eye of the philosopher, as well as insights into how better to bring medical practice in line with patient experiences."

We agree with some objections of Gergel and Sholl, disagree with some and others do not relate to our study. We start with this latter group which includes just point (a). We don't feel affected by point (a) in the sense that we have never intended this study as a critique at evidence-based medicine in MS care. Although it might be true that some phenomenologists associate themselves with 'complementary' and 'alternative' medicine (Waksler, 2001), we do not nor wish to contest the proper place of the natural sciences in medicine. Thus the idea that the critique of Sholl that phenomenology misrepresents the viewpoints of naturalism (casually defined by Gergel as "the objective measure of biological dysfunction") does not apply to our study.

With other objections we agree but we believe that we have managed to incorporate them in an appreciate way in the design of our study. We correspond with point (b) in the sense that we consider the distinction between "normal" and "pathological" as problematic since it is within phenomenology undecidable which category applies when. Therefore we side in the issue of the relationship between "normal" and "pathological" rather with Carel (2013) than with Toombs who defined illness as *disruption* of the (normal) unity between self, body and world. However

Carel situates illness as a *limit case* of (normal) embodied experience: "Illness sheds light on normal experience, revealing its ordinary and thus overlooked structure. Illness produces a distancing effect, which allows us to observe normal human and cognition via their pathological counterpart" (p. 345).

Firstly, regarding the objections related to insight (1) we mention that we have not adopted an individualistic stance towards lived experience. Rather we emphasize phenomenology as an intersubjective endeavor. We conceived therefore the research interview as a relational scene of address that functioned as the intersubjective correlate for the events that where originally experienced as an individual. Also we maintained the idea of relationships as horizons to human experience. We therefore think that the accusation of phenomenology as an ultimately solipsist endeavor doesn't apply to our study.

Secondly, regarding the objections that refer to insight (2) we maintain that in our design there is not a separation between pre-existing assumptions (that must be suspended during the process of phenomenological reduction) and isolated and pure understanding of phenomena (like illness). We agree with Gergel that such a divide is actually impossible. Contextualization entails eliciting a lived experience as an element of a subjective lifeworld from which it gains its meaning. In our study the process of reduction entails hence not the suspension of the context of a phenomenon but rather of the appreciation of the relation between the phenomenon and the context that supplies for its significance.

Thirdly, regarding the objections related to insight (3) we agree with Gergel that phenomenology sometimes doesn't address the intertwining of the self and the lived body in a satisfactory way. We also agree with Gergel that the complex relation between the body and the self is in need of further research. In the design of our study we managed this issue by adopting an adapted version of IPA. In this version the issue of embodied subjectivity as a dynamic and complex phenomenon is explicitly and to our mind properly addressed.

Finally regarding the objections related to insight (4) we again agree with Gergel that many accounts of phenomenology aren't well defined and almost indistinct from any other humanistic approach to medicine. We believe to have managed this issue by making a careful distinction between phenomenology as a moral approach to care (backgrounded by ethics of care) and as a method for qualitative research. However we passionately disagree with Gergel when she writes that "the poles of the opposition, however we wish to name it – biomedical and humanistic, orthodox and radical, are not nearly so clear or entrenched as phenomenologists might suggest" (p. 1107). Of course it is true that science becomes continually more equipped to define the unique biomedical and psychological 'fingerprint' that each individual carries. But we think that this 'fingerprint' never account for the unique phenomenon of subjectivity such as it emerges from first person accounts (of illness) and other individual (and collective) demonstrations of human creativity and freedom.

Lessons learned from a phenomenological ethics of care

We now complete this section with a discussion of what can be learned from our attempt to create a phenomenological ethics of care for people recently diagnosed with MS. We embarked on this enterprise because we wanted to understand what it means for people to have to go through the experience of living with MS and to see how these experiences are rooted in their relational and (occasionally) political contexts (Casterlé et al., 2011; Klaver et al., 2013). Concerning the relational context of people, the lived experiences of relationships of the participants of this study presents a mixed picture. Some participants found themselves (after a while) back in a closer relationship with respectively their mother (P3), parents in law (P5), father (P6), brother (P7), or husband (P8). But relationships appeared also to be thwarted by illness. Illness threatened cherished ideas about falling in love and having a romantic relationship (P3). It menaced expectations about how to be a good parent (P1, P7, P9), a good partner (P4, P8) and a caretaker for parents in old age (P10). And although some participants tried to find (medical) professionals they could relate to (for example P10), some of them also perceived contacts with (medical) professionals partly a necessary evil (P10) or just as a way to get something they wanted (P4).

We haven't found in the body of literature in ethics of care any descriptions of lived experiences (of patients with MS) of relationships that resonate with the mixed picture that emerged out of the lived experiences of relationships of the participants of this study. To our best knowledge the one and only description of case of a person with MS in the body of literature of ethics of care presents a lot less ambiguous picture of lived relationships. This case was presented by first generation ethicist of care Kittay, during a lecture that she gave in 2010 at February 3rd in Bologna (Kittay, 2011). In this lecture, Kittay stages, as illustration of the purpose of her ethics of care, the story of comedian and MS patient Richard Pryor (1940-2005). Kittay commented in that lecture on an interview that Pryor had given at 27 October 2000 for the U.S. National Public Radio (NPR) at the occasion of the release of the complete edition of his recordings:[22]

> "[Pryor] said that as he lost old capacities, he had to learn new ones; that the Multiple Sclerosis was in fact 'the best thing that had ever happened to me.' The incredulity of the interviewer was palpable. Then Pryor explained that he had lived a life in which he had felt he could never trust anyone. Because, in order to walk from one end of a room to the other, a person must depend on another, he learned how to trust for the first time in his life. This, he replied, was the best thing that ever happened to him. [*Kittay concludes*:] The trust that Pryor had to learn when he became disabled[23] – and the need for trustworthiness that warrants such trust – ought to be a feature of all our lives."

When we compare the Pryor case with the lived experiences the 10 participants of our study, the difference is evident. Pryor told how he had learned, forced by the progression of MS, to develop, for the first time, relationships of trust. Pryor's message has become, after 14 years of living with MS, unambiguous: getting MS has been a good thing for him. This unambiguity contrasts with the mixed picture that emerged from the lived experiences of relationships of the participants. How should we understand this difference? The point of a phenomenological study can't be the determination whether an account of a phenomenon is 'right' or 'wrong'. Rather a phenomenological study should present and enhance the richness of the phenomenon as lived (Patton, 2005) and establish how it adds up to our understanding of the phenomenon.

---

[22] A recording of this interview is available at the site of National Public Radio (NPR): http://www.npr.org/templates/story/story.php?storyId=1113112 (accessed at September 30, 2016). Also interesting is an undated audio recording of a show in which Pryor discusses his illness (including a funny account of his contacts with physicians) which is available at YouTube: https://youtu.be/OJLOLSV43YQ (accessed at September 30, 2016).
[23] Pryor was diagnosed with MS in 1986, according to "The Official Biography of Richard Pryor, (http://richardpryor.com/biography.php", accessed at December 14, 2016).

When we use this more appropriate angle to evaluate the contribution of our phenomenological investigation to ethics of care, we think that our findings on lived relationships complement the current understanding of relationships in ethics of care, by the suggestion that *lived* (moral significance of) relationships and dependencies have *degrees of intensity*. Viewed from the perspective of "degrees of intensity", the Pryor case presents an instance wherein the moral significance ("best thing that had ever happened to me") of living with others in a asymmetric relationship is maximally felt. The participants of our study, however, lived relationships and illness less unambiguously. Sometimes they expressed lived relationships and illness even as a way of *suffering* (Toombs, 1988). One can speculate about to what extent persons recently diagnosed with MS can learn, like Pryor, over time, a new understanding wherein illness is understood as a genuine possibility for a good life. But perhaps more importantly – and more proper for phenomenological study with a background in ethics of care – it is to ask what recommendations follow from this study for people that want to *help* people with recently diagnosed MS (professional and informal provers of care alike).

In sum, we suggest, based on our research, that a consistent phenomenological approach provides a broader analytical lens, through which to understand the lived experience of patients and establish them with a certain amount of rigor. The layers of intensity offer points of orientation for care and they curb any potential and hidden moral vision that may be lurking beneath the theories or practice of care. The imperative is to connect with the patient's subjective experience and support them in that experience, not according to a normative prescription of how life should be lived but according to how life is actually experienced by the patients in the here and now.

Recommendations: important focuses

First we turn to our recommendations for medical professionals. Our analysis of patients' lived experience of the process of diagnosis presented a picture of patients being challenged by physical complaints with potentially life threatening implications. From the patient perspective these complaints are then investigated – sometimes after a while but sometimes also instantaneously – in an alien environment with strange instruments that are operated by strangers. The gap between what is at stake (virtually everything) and the familiarity with the involved medical professionals and applied procedures (almost none) is massive. This is something that medical professionals can account for, verbally or attitudinally, in their contacts with patients during testing for MS. Even modest acknowledgement of the precarity of the situation of being tested for MS might help patients to regain a certain degree of control and confidence. Similarly lived experiences of using disease modifying therapies (DMT's) showed that the establishment and continuation of the practice of taking (initially strange and unknown) medications is from the patient perspective perilous and a relational rather than individual affair. Medical professionals can account for such experiences by recognizing tacitly and perhaps sometimes also openly that shared decision making in taking DMT's includes sometimes not only the doctor and the patient but also his or her close relatives.

Second, and lastly, we turn to recommendations for those who are usually described as informal care givers (often close relatives) and people who work as professionals with people with recently diagnosed MS that have paid jobs. Lived experiences of MS within the social structure of families presents a mixed picture. Sometimes relationships were felt to have become more solid. At other instances participants became aware of illness as a present or future threat for the relationships with their most loved ones. It seems that people with recently diagnosed MS care a great deal about sustaining and safe relationships with close others. Verbal and attitudinal assurance by informal care givers and or close relatives (parents, partners, children, brothers and sisters) to patients of ongoing commitment and trustworthiness (Kittay, 2011) seems to be a good way to address experiences of loneliness and uncertainty that can emerge in patients while living with illness in families. People that work as professionals with people with recently diagnosed MS can learn from lived experiences related to paid work that work means for people (with MS) a lot more than just earning money for living. Bureaucratic procedures surrounding sick leave and early retirement are extensive and the financial stakes, especially for smaller employers, are high. The risk of disappearance from view of the employee as a person, for which work is personally and socially meaningful, seems to be high. The accounts of the participants of this study about keeping and losing paid work may help professionals that help people with illnesses to avoid that risk.

A final note

Several times in this study the suggestion was raised that the improvement of professional care in MS could also entail the cultivation (Toombs 2001) of a habit of mind (Greenfield 2010) for professionals that is aware of illness and care such as they are lived by patients. One could of course embark on this cultivation on an individual basis by reading books, listening to music, experiencing art and watching movies referring to health, illness and corporality. For us, for example, a huge source for inspiration during the development of this dissertation was the true story of *Elle* journalist Jean-Dominique Bauby (as staged in the 2007 biographical drama film *Le Scaphandre et le Papillon*, The Diving Bell and the Butterfly) that depicts – from his own perspective – his life after suffering a massive stroke at the age of 43. But we suggest that the cultivation of a more holistic and inclusive perspective on illness and care could also be stimulated on a *collective* basis. Meetings of physicians, MS nurses, and patients to share the latest developments in MS research have become common in recent years. One could imagine comparable platforms being created to exchange fine-art photography (Bolaki, 2016), books, music, art and movies about illness and care as first-person phenomena in the lives of providers and receivers of care. We think that such platforms may help to get the critical insights of phenomenology out of the dusty academic cabinets were they usually reside and into hospitals' and patients' homes. The emergence of true and strong *mixed* relational networks of patients and MS professionals might be enhanced by experiencing and discussing art together. This may even have beneficial effects on the meetings in the consultation and examination rooms of the hospital. There the topic of the meeting might not only be the disease but also the illness such as patient and physician might have previously explored them together at meetings revolving around illness and care not as topics of natural science but as problems of *Geist* and *Leben* (Husserl, 1965).

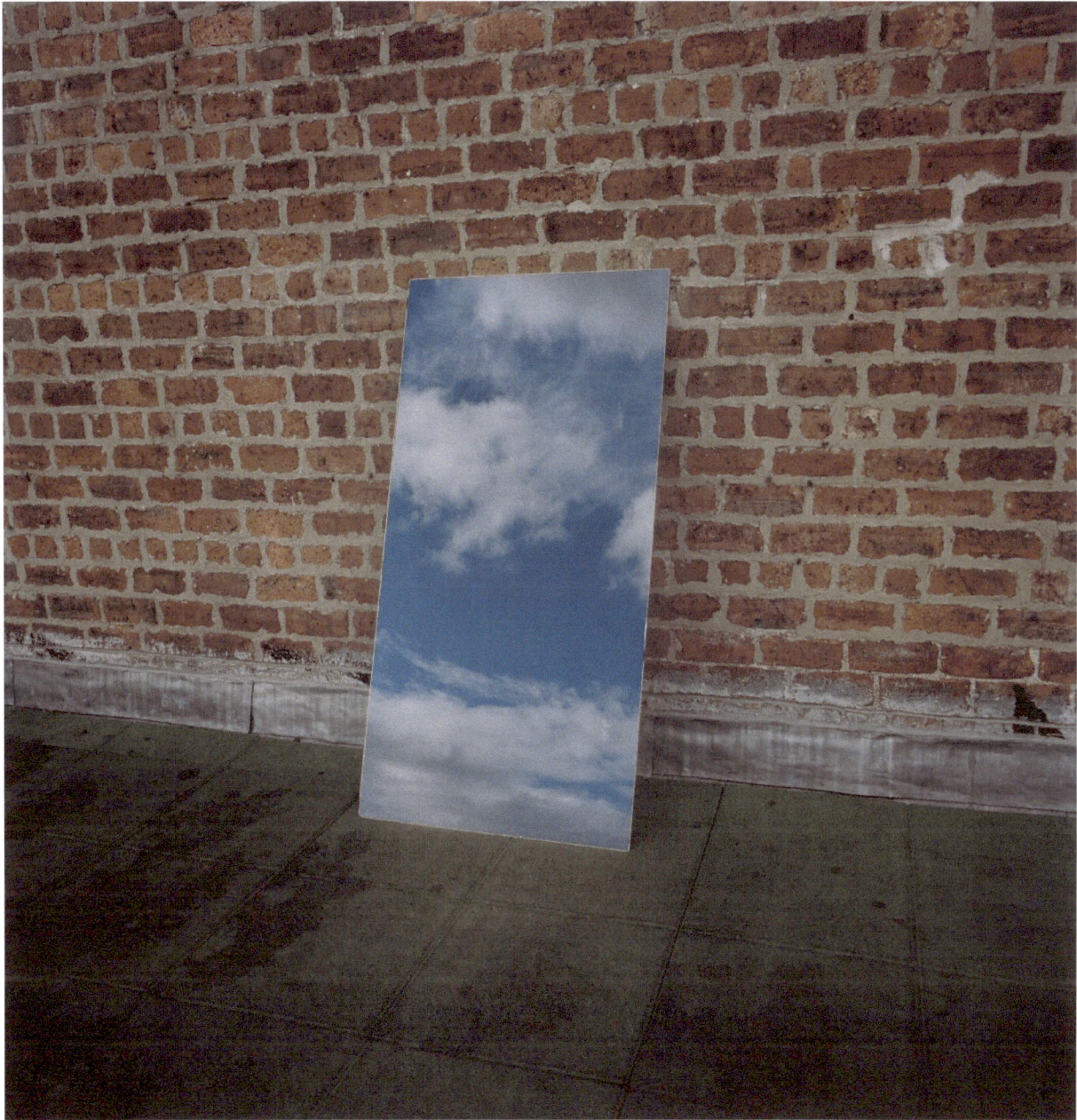

Appendix to chapter 1: Breaking bad news, how to make the difference

After European Journal for Person Centered Healthcare *had accepted our article* "Developing Patient-Centred Care for Multiple Sclerosis (MS). Learning from Patient Perspectives on the process of MS diagnosis", *its editor-in-chief, Prof. Andrew Miles MSc MPhil PhD DSc (hc), invited Dr. Marianne van Iersel MD, a clinical specialist in geriatric medicine, to write an editorial about it. This editorial will appear together with our article in this journal.*

Van Iersel, Marianne van (2016) Breaking bad news, how to make the difference. European Journal for Person Centered Healthcare 4 (4) doi: 10.5750/ejpch.v4i4.1265.

Breaking bad news represents an important moment in the diagnostic process and is generally recognised as a core professional skill that physicians have to master. Accordingly, it's incorporated in communication training of medical students and residents and fills complete chapters in communication teaching books (Buckman, 2010). In medical training it is a separate entrusted professional activity (EPA) to ensure that it receives particular attention and assessment. Despite all the attention to teach and train this skill, it still proves to be a difficult , a moment prone to mistakes and miscommunication (Hanratty et al., 2011).

Part of the problem is the emotional state of the patient at the moment of disclose. The uncertainty, fears, discomfort and symptoms can make it harder to grasp the message the way it is intended. This is understandable and can only be partially influenced. To improve understanding and decrease misperceptions and doubts afterwards a few aspects of breaking bad news deserve extra attention.

The moment of diagnostic disclosure is a distinct moment, but foremost embedded in the whole diagnostic and therapeutic process. It cannot be separated from the complete process. For example, a technically correct performed disclose of the diagnosis cannot make up for omissions in personal contact in the preceding trajectory. A 'good' disclosure of the diagnosis of a debilitating disease also requires empathy and translation of the general concept to personal problems, risks and options. Let us consider first the trajectory before the disclose and then look at empathy.

To individualise the diagnosis it requires personalised medicine in the true sense of the word. It requires weighing of individual preferences and personal circumstances. Obviously, personal preferences differ between patients (De Ceuninck van Capelle et al., 2016a). They depend on previous experiences, personality, the disease trajectory so far and individual fears. Because the relation between patient and physician is not equal, it requires active investigation by the physician to discover patient preferences and to know how a diagnosis would influences the patient's life. The varying pattern in the presentations of signs and symptoms of multiple sclerosis (MS) can make the period of uncertainty between first symptoms and the diagnosis quite long as it can take some time to develop and comply to the diagnostic criteria. This makes the decision about how and when to break the bad news more difficult. De Ceuninck van Capelle et al. (2016a) showed that a direct disclose of the diagnosis MS is only possible with behold of trust if patient and physician know each other already. In other cases it's preferable to start with a discussion of options and go from there. However, the interviewed patients reported that these methods were not always followed through. Other authors also showed a difference between preferences of patients and clinical practice. For example, most patients, 90%, prefer to receive information about the disease and prognosis of MS during the diagnostic trajectory of their first signs and symptoms (Messina et al., 2015). Ninety-one percent also prefers to hear the diagnosis MS. However, this only happens in 44% of all trajectories. It not only doesn't suit the patient preferences, it also hampers patient participation in disease management and decreases the trust felt in the neurologist (Papathanasopoulos et al., 2008; Papathanasopoulos, Nikolakopoulou, & Scolding, 2005). Most diagnostic disclosures happen in private settings and family members are present in 69%. The most important preferences of patients regarding diagnostic disclosure are enough time and a disclosure tailored to the patients profile, some follow-up with a psychologist or patient group meeting to assimilate with the diagnosis.

Empathy The term 'empathy' receives a lot of attention in the surveys and interviews. Most patients can recall the moment of receiving the diagnosis: they have a clear memory of how the message had been told and if they had felt empathy. In many cases empathy matters more than the exact words or presentation of facts. Empathy can be expressed verbal and nonverbal. Verbally empathy can be shown trough the words chosen in disclosing the diagnosis and addressing the (un)correctness of the patients worst nightmares. The nonverbal aspect of feeling empathy is large. Crucial aspects are a physician who shows its trustworthiness by being on time, well-prepared and behaves interested. When patients feel the good intentions and empathy, the exact words matter less.

Physicians acknowledge the importance of showing empathy. It is one of the key elements that makes a technically good physician outstanding (Boerebach et al., 2014; Lombarts et al., 2014). To be able to express empathy requires a state of being, being in the moment instead of somewhere else and on the run with a list of tasks in mind. It requires openness, the effort of trying to be near and involved. Despite that caring for patients is the main reason to become a physician, to stay as involved and empathic as starting students and physicians proves difficult for a subgroup. It's not that this subgroup want to be harsh or rude. It's more about barriers to show the desired behaviour. And of these barriers there are a lot. Time constrains are often one of the first arguments physicians mention. Time is money, also in health care. Physicians have to see a certain amount of patient to fulfil the 'production' goal of the organisation. Second, although patient care should be the core business, many other tasks also ask time. Killing for basic contact and empathy is if patients feel the physician is in a hurry and has no or not enough time for them. In these circumstances the adagio counts: the quicker you want to go as a physician, the slower the process gets.

How much time a physician has for appointments is often out of his/her reach and dictated by the organisation. It requires clear priorities to organise care processes around the patient and according to important moments in the process. Processes should be organised in a way that patients and physicians had had time to know each other prior to the diagnostic disclosure. This facilitates not only for patients but also for the messengers of the bad news the task is easier: to bring a serious diagnosis without a clue how to do it sensibly for that particular patient is a nightmare. Even with the best of intentions and organisation communication can go wrong. To tune in with the expectations, questions and fears of patients also requires sensitivity to cultural matters and values of patients and oneself. Last, it can be emotionally draining to break bad news many times a day. How to do so, find balance and refresh energy is up to the individual physician.

All above is what the physician should do and what the patients prefer. But what are the roles of the patients themselves and the organisation to reach those goals? As De Ceuninck van Capelle et al. (2016a) already described, patients can take several roles: from passive to consumer or an active citizen who actively participates in shared decision making. Active participation in choices sounds great, but to perform like this in severely distressing situations as in to await results and a possibly devastating diagnosis, requires a lot. In daily practice many patients follow without many objections the hospital routine. Public campaigns try to make patients as well prepared as possible, for example to let them makes list of important questions to ask the physician. With the internet patients can gather a lot of information themselves. How and what type of information had been found also influences the process of diagnostic disclosure. This aspects haven't been reported on in diagnostic disclosure studies. Other sources of information and patient empowerment can be the patients groups. These peers can help in preparing questions for meetings with the physician and give some of the so needed emotional support.

As already mentioned before, part of the comments regarding diagnostic disclosure refer to organisation of care. The requests of the patients sound simple: Not too much time between investigation and results (although some time to get adjusted that bad news probably is coming of help) and a clear indication of waiting times for test results and appointments. With the addition that the perception of time by patients is different and most often a lot longer than that of health care workers. Furthermore, where one patient has one to a few health care workers, a physician sees many patients a day. In daily practice the points named above prove hard to realise, although technical novelties in logistic and planning systems are promising. In many cases the planning of appointments is process instead of patient centred. Other organisational challenges are to keep all other people involved in the care of that patient well-informed, such as a general practitioner and physiotherapist.

Breaking bad news in other diseases MS is not the only disease that forewarns a disabling disease with an unpredictable course. It's interesting to know if the experience of the diagnostic disclosure is different for other diseases. Examples of more or less life threatening diseases with possible debilitating consequences are breast cancer and dementia. Patients with these diseases showed similar preferences and experiences as noted by De Ceuninck van Capelle et al. (2016a). They also differ in their preferences how they would have liked to receive the diagnosis and the importance of the relationship with their physician (Lecouturier et al., 2008; Samsi et al., 2014). For example Attai, Hampton, Staley, Borgert, & Landercasper (2016) found large differences between actual an preferred care in the mode of communication of the diagnosis breast cancer and waiting time for test results. Only 50% received the preferred mode of communication of the diagnosis. This first communication was only in 39% face-to-face, although some preferred the telephone or electronic modes with an appointment afterwards. Although the authors held a survey in a specific population with mainly Caucasian, well-educated women, their preferences are similar to the MS patients: timely appointments and patient-specific modes of communication. Furthermore, results are highly congruent between surveys, interviews and expert panels.

Thus, the diagnostic disclosure marks an important moment in the diagnostic process and is a good start to discuss and design a personal treatment plan. As a physician you only have one chance to break the bad news as sensibly as you can: go for it and use all information sources available to individualise the message. I can only but agree with the plea of De Ceuninck van Capelle et al. (2016a) to let patient and physician make the diagnostic journey together, so patient perspectives on the disease and preferences of the diagnostic disclosure are known and showing empathy fits in so much more naturally.

References

Ashworth, P. D. (2006). Seeing oneself as a carer in the activity of caring: Attending to the lifeworld of a person with Alzheimer's disease. *International Journal of Qualitative Studies on Health and Well-being*, *1*(4), 212–225.

Attai, D. J., Hampton, R., Staley, A. C., Borgert, A., & Landercasper, J. (2016). What Do Patients Prefer? Understanding Patient Perspectives on Receiving a New Breast Cancer Diagnosis. *Annals of Surgical Oncology*, *23*(10), 3182–3189.

Audhoe, S. S., Hoving, J. L., Sluiter, J. K., & Frings-Dresen, M. H. (2010). Vocational interventions for unemployed: effects on work participation and mental distress. A systematic review. *Journal of occupational rehabilitation*, *20*(1), 1–13.

Audulv, Å., Packer, T., & Versnel, J. (2014). Identifying gaps in knowledge: A map of the qualitative literature concerning life with a neurological condition. *Chronic Illness*, *10*(3), 192–243.

Baart, A., Vosman, F. J. H., & others. (2015). *De patient terug van weggeweest: Werken aan Menslievende zorg in het ziekenhuis*. Amsterdam: SWP.

Barker-Collo, S., Cartwright, C., & Read, J. (2006). Into the unknown: The experiences of individuals living with multiple sclerosis. *Journal of Neuroscience Nursing*, *38*(6), 435–446.

Barry, M. J., & Edgman-Levitan, S. (2012). Shared decision making—the pinnacle of patient-centered care. *New England Journal of Medicine*, *366*(9), 780–781.

Bevan, M. T. (2014). A Method of Phenomenological Interviewing. *Qualitative Health Research*, *24*(1), 136–144.

Boerebach, B. C., Scheepers, R. A., Leeuw, R. M. van der, Heineman, M. J., Arah, O. A., & Lombarts, K. M. (2014). The impact of clinicians' personality and their interpersonal behaviors on the quality of patient care: a systematic review. *International Journal for Quality in Health Care*, *26*(4), 426–481.

Bolaki, S. (2016). Capturing the worlds of multiple sclerosis: Hannah Laycock's photography. *Medical Humanities*, medhum–2016.

Brandes, D. W., Callender, T., Lathi, E., & O'Leary, S. (2008). A review of disease-modifying therapies for MS: maximizing adherence and minimizing adverse events. *Current Medical Research and Opinion, 25*(1), 77–92.

Buckman, R. (2010). *Practical plans for difficult conversations in medicine: Strategies that work in breaking bad news*. Baltimore, MD: Johns Hopkins University Press.

Burnfield, A. (1984). Doctor-patient dilemmas in multiple sclerosis. *Journal of medical ethics, 10*(1), 21–26.

Carel, H. (2012). Phenomenology as a resource for patients. *Journal of Medicine and Philosophy, 37*(2), 96–113.

Carel, H. H. (2013). Illness, phenomenology, and philosophical method. *Theoretical medicine and bioethics, 34*(4), 345–357.

Casterlé, B. D. de, Verhaeghe, S. T., Kars, M. C., Coolbrandt, A., Stevens, M., Stubbe, M., Deweirdt, N., et al. (2011). Researching lived experience in health care: Significance for care ethics. *Nursing ethics, 18*(2), 232–242.

Ceuninck van Capelle, Archie de; Visser, Leo H.; Vosman, F. J. H. (2015). Multiple Sclerosis and Work: An Interpretative Phenomenological Analysis of the Perspective of Persons with early stage MS. *Journal of Multiple Sclerosis, 2:4*. doi:10.4172/2376-0389.1000158.

Ceuninck van Capelle, Archie de; Visser, Leo H.; Vosman, F. J. H. (2016a). Developing Patient-Centred Care for Multiple Sclerosis (MS): Learning from Patient Perspectives on the process of MS diagnosis. *European Journal for Person Centered Healthcare, 4*(4). doi: 10.5750/ejpch.v4i4.1191.

Ceuninck van Capelle, Archie de; Visser, Leo H.; Vosman, F. J. H. (2016b). Multiple Sclerosis (MS) in the Life Cycle of the Family: An Interpretative Phenomenological Analysis of the Perspective of

Persons With Recently Diagnosed MS. *Families, Systems, & Health*. doi: 10.1037/fsh0000216.

Compston, A., & Coles, A. (2008). Multiple sclerosis. *The Lancet, 372*(9648), 1502–1517.

Costello, K., Halper, J., Kalb, R., Skutnik, L., & Rapp, R. (2016). The use of disease-modifying therapies in multiple sclerosis. Principles and current evidence. A consensus paper by the multiple sclerosis coalition.

Creswell, J. W. (1998). Qualitative inquiry and research design: Choosing among five designs. Thousand Oaks, CA: Sage.

Crouch, M., & McKenzie, H. (2006). The logic of small samples in interview-based qualitative research. *Social science information, 45*(4), 483–499.

Dahlberg, K., Todres, L., & Galvin, K. (2009). Lifeworld-led healthcare is more than patient-led care: An existential view of well-being. *Medicine, Health Care and Philosophy, 12*(3), 265–271.

De Rijk, A., Janssen, N., Van Lierop, B., Alexanderson, K., & Nijhuis, F. (2009). A behavioral approach to RTW after sickness absence: the development of instruments for the assessment of motivational determinants, motivation and key actors' attitudes. *Work: A Journal of Prevention, Assessment and Rehabilitation, 33*(3), 273–285.

Dejours, C., & Deranty, J.-P. (2010). The centrality of work. *Critical Horizons: A Journal of Philosophy & Social Theory, 11*(2), 167–180.

Dejours, C., & Gernet, I. (2012). Work, Subjectivity and Trust [Travail, subjectivité et confiance]. *Nouvelle revue de psychosociologie*, (1), 75–91.

Dekkers, W. J. (1995). FJJ Buytendijk's concept of an anthropological physiology. *Theoretical Medicine, 16*(1), 15–39.

Dennison, L., Smith, E. M., Bradbury, K., & Galea, I. (2016). How Do People with Multiple Sclerosis Experience Prognostic Uncertainty and Prognosis Communication? A Qualitative Study. *PloS one, 11*(7), e0158982, doi: 10.1371/journal.pone.0158982.

Dennison, L., Yardley, L., Devereux, A., & Moss-Morris, R. (2010). Experiences of adjusting to early stage Multiple Sclerosis. *Journal of health psychology*, doi: 10.1177/1359105310384299.

Derwenskus, J. (2011). Current Disease-Modifying Treatment of Multiple Sclerosis. *Mount Sinai Journal of Medicine: A Journal of Translational and Personalized Medicine, 78*(2), 161–175.

Detaille, S. I., Gulden, J. W. van der, Engels, J. A., Heerkens, Y. F., & Dijk, F. J. van. (2010). Using intervention mapping (IM) to develop a self-management programme for employees with a chronic disease in the Netherlands. *BMC Public Health, 10*(1), 353-364.

Dyck, I. (1995). Hidden geographies: The changing lifeworlds of women with multiple sclerosis. *Social science & medicine, 40*(3), 307–320.

Dyck, I., & Jongbloed, L. (2000). Women with multiple sclerosis and employment issues: A focus on social and institutional environments. *Canadian Journal of Occupational Therapy, 67*(5), 337–346.

Eijk, M. van der Faber, M., Shamma S. Al, Munneke, M. , Bloem, B. R. (2011). Moving towards patient-centered healthcare for patients with Parkinson's disease. *Parkinsonism and Related Disorders* 17, 360-364.

Elian, M., & Dean, G. (1985). To tell or not to tell the diagnosis of multiple sclerosis. *The Lancet, 326*(8445), 27–28.

Evans, C., Marrie, R. A., Zhu, F., Leung, S., Lu, X., Melesse, D. Y., Kingwell, E., et al. (2016). Adherence and persistence to drug therapies for multiple sclerosis: A population-based study. *Multiple Sclerosis and Related Disorders, 8,* 78–85.

Finlay, L. (2003). The intertwining of body, self and world: A phenomenological study of living with recently-diagnosed multiple sclerosis. *Journal of Phenomenological Psychology, 34*(2), 157–178.

Fisher, P. (2007). Experiential knowledge challenges 'normality'and individualized citizenship: towards 'another way of being'. *Disability & Society, 22*(3), 283–298.

Franche, R.-L., & Krause, N. (2002). Readiness for return to work following injury or illness: conceptualizing the interpersonal impact of health care, workplace, and insurance factors. *Journal of occupational rehabilitation, 12*(4), 233–256.

Frank, A. W. (2000). The standpoint of storyteller. *Qualitative health research, 10*(3), 354–365.

Fuchs, T. (2000). *Leib, Raum, Person: Entwurf einer phänomenologischen Anthropologie.* Stuttgart: Klett-Cotta.

Gastmans, C. (2006). The care perspective in healthcare ethics. *Essentials of teaching and learning in nursing ethics: Perspectives and methods,* 135–148.

Gergel, T. L. (2012). Medicine and the individual: Is phenomenology the answer? *Journal of Evaluation in Clinical Practice, 18*(5), 1102–1109.

Gerteis, M. (1993). *Through the patient's eyes: understanding and promoting patient-centered care.* Jossey Bass.

Glaser, B. G., & Strauss, A. L. (2009). *The discovery of grounded theory: Strategies for qualitative research.* New Brunswick, NJ: Transaction Publishers.

Greenfield, B., & Jensen, G. M. (2010). Beyond a code of ethics: Phenomenological ethics for everyday practice. *Physiotherapy Research International, 15*(2), 88–95.

Grypdonck, M. (1997). Die Bedeutung qualitativer Forschung für die Pflegekunde und die Pflegewissen-schaft. *Pflege, 10*(4), 222–228.

Grytten, N., & Måseide, P. (2006). 'When I am together with them I feel more ill.' The stigma of multiple sclerosis experienced in social relationships. *Chronic Illness, 2*(3), 195–208.

Guest, G., Bunce, A., & Johnson, L. (2006). How many interviews are enough? An experiment with data saturation and variability. *Field methods, 18*(1), 59–82.

Hal, L. B. van, Meershoek, A., Rijk, A. de, & Nijhuis, F. (2012). Going beyond vocational rehabilitation as a training of skills: return-to-work as an identity issue. *Disability & Society, 27*(1), 81–93.

Halper, J. (2008). Comprehensive care in multiple sclerosis–a patient-centred approach. *European Neuro-logical Review, 3*, 72–4.

Hanratty, B., Lowson, E., Holmes, L., Grande, G., Jacoby, A., Payne, S., Seymour, J., et al. (2011). Breaking bad news sensitively: What is important to patients in their last year of life? *BMJ supportive & palliative care, 2*(1), 24-28.

Hansen, K., Schüssel, K., Kieble, M., Werning, J., Schulz, M., Friis, R., Pöhlau, D., et al. (2015). Adherence to disease modifying drugs among patients with multiple sclerosis in germany: A retrospective cohort study. *PloS one, 10*(7), e0133279, doi: 10.1371/journal.pone.o133279.

Hartmann, M., Bäzner, E., Wild, B., Eisler, I., & Herzog, W. (2010). Effects of interventions involving the family in the treatment of adult patients with chronic physical diseases: A meta-analysis. *Psycho-therapy and psychosomatics, 79*(3), 136–148.

Heier, J., Kohlen, H., & Olthuis, G. (2014). *Moral Boundaries Redrawn: The Significance of Joan Tronto's Argument for Political Theory, Professional Ethics, and Care As Practice*. Leuven: Peeters Publishers.

Heijst, A. van. (2011). *Professional loving care: An ethical view of the health care sector*. Leuven: Peeters Publishers.

Hodge, N. (2008). Evaluating Lifeworld as an emancipatory methodology. *Disability & Society, 23*(1), 29–40.

Holmes, D., Kennedy, S. L., & Perron, A. (2004). The mentally ill and social exclusion: A critical examination of the use of seclusion from the patient's perspective. *Issues in mental health nursing, 25*(6), 559–578.

Holmes, D., Murray, S. J., & Knack, N. (2015). Experiencing seclusion in a forensic psychiatric setting: A phenomenological study. *Journal of forensic nursing, 11*(4), 200–213.

Holmes, D., Murray, S. J., Perron, A., & Rail, G. (2006). Deconstructing the evidence-based discourse in health sciences: Truth, power and fascism. *International Journal of Evidence-Based Healthcare, 4*(3), 180–186.

Hunter, S. (2016). Overview and diagnosis of multiple sclerosis. *The American journal of managed care, 22*(6), S141-S150.

Husserl, E. (1965). *Phenomenology and the Crisis of Philosophy: Philosophy as a Rigorous Science, and Philosophy and the Crisis of European Man*. New York, N.Y.: Harper & Row.

Iersel, M. van (2016). Breaking bad news, how to make the difference. *European Journal for Person Centered Healthcare, 4*(4). doi: 10.5750/ejpch.v4i4.1265.

Institute of Medicine (2001). *Crossing the quality chasm: A new health system for the 21st century*. Washington, DC: National Academy Press.

Jason, A. W., Niederhauser, V., Marshburn, D., LaVela, S.L. (2014). Defining patient experience. *Patient Experience Journal, 1*(1), 7–19.

Johnson, K. L., Kuehn, C. M., Yorkston, K. M., Kraft, G. H., Klasner, E., & Amtmann, D. (2006). Patient perspectives on disease-modifying therapy in multiple sclerosis. *International Journal of MS Care, 8*(1), 11–18.

Johnson, K. L., Yorkston, K. M., Klasner, E. R., Kuehn, C. M., Johnson, E., & Amtmann, D. (2004). The cost and benefits of employment: A qualitative study of experiences of persons with multiple sclerosis. *Archives of Physical Medicine and Rehabilation, 85*(2), 201–209.

Julian, L. J., Vella, L., Vollmer, T., Hadjimichael, O., & Mohr, D. C. (2008). Employment in multiple sclerosis. *Journal of Neurology, 255*(9), 1354–1360.

Kittay, E. F. (2011). The Ethics of Care, Dependence, and Disability. *Ratio Juris, 24*(1), 49–58.

Klaver, K., Elst, E. van, & Baart, A. J. (2013). Demarcation of the ethics of care as a discipline: Discussion article. *Nursing Ethics*, doi: 10.1177/0969733013500162.

Kohlen, H. (2011). Care transformations: attentiveness, professional ethics and thoughts towards differentiation. *Nursing Ethics 18*(2), 258-261.

Koopman, W., & Schweitzer, A. (1999). The journey to multiple sclerosis: A qualitative study. *Journal of Neuroscience Nursing, 31*(1), 17–26.

Krahn, T. M. (2014). Care ethics for guiding the process of multiple sclerosis diagnosis. *Journal of medical ethics*, 802–806.

Krause, N., & Ragland, D. R. (1994). Occupational disability due to low back pain: A new interdisciplinary classification based on a phase model of disability. *Spine, 19*(9), 1011–1020.

Kremer, A., Wevers, C., & Andries, F. (1997). *Werken met multiple sclerose*. Amsterdam: NIA TNO.

Lage, M., Castelli-Haley, J., & Oleen-Burkey, M. (2005). Effect of immunomodulatory therapy and other factors on employment loss time in multiple sclerosis. *Work, 27*(2), 143–151.

Le Guillant, L. (1984). *Quelle psychiatrie pour notre temps?* Toulouse: Érès.

Lecouturier, J., Bamford, C., Hughes, J. C., Francis, J. J., Foy, R., Johnston, M., & Eccles, M. P. (2008). Appropriate disclosure of a diagnosis of dementia: Identifying the key behaviours of 'best practice'. *BMC Health Services Research*, doi: 10.1186/1472-6963-8-95.

Levine, C. (1983). Delaying the diagnosis: Truth-telling and multiple sclerosis. *The Hastings Center Report, 13*(3), 2-3.

Lombarts, K. M., Plochg, T., Thompson, C. A., Arah, O. A., Consortium, Duq. P., & others. (2014). Measuring professionalism in medicine and nursing: Results of a European survey. *PloS one, 9*(5), e97069, doi: 10.1371/journal.pone.0097069.

Lorig, K. R., & Holman, H. R. (2003). Self-management education: History, definition, outcomes, and mechanisms. *Annals of Behavioral Medicine, 26*(1), 1–7.

Lowden, D., Lee, V., & Ritchie, J. A. (2014). Redefining Self: Patients' Decision Making About Treatment for Multiple Sclerosis. *Journal of Neuroscience Nursing, 46*(4), E14–E24.

Martin, J. L. (2011). *The explanation of social action*. Oxford: Oxford University Press.

Martinsen, E. (2011). Harm in the absence of care: Towards a medical ethics that cares. *Nursing ethics*, *18*(2), 174–183.

Martinsen, E. H. (2011). Care for Nurses Only? Medicine and the Perceiving Eye. *Health Care Analysis*, *19*(1), 15–27.

Martinsen, E. H., & Solbakk, J. H. (2012). Illness as a condition of our existence in the world: On illness and pathic existence. *Medical humanities*, *38*(1), 44–49.

Mason, M. (2010). Sample size and saturation in PhD studies using qualitative interviews. *Forum Qualitative Sozialforschung/Forum: Qualitative Social Research, 11*(3), 1-13.

Mattson, D. H. (2002). Alphabet soup: A personal, evolving, mostly evidence-based and logical, sequential approach to the "ABCNR" drugs in multiple sclerosis. *Seminars in neurology, 22*(1), 17–25.

McDonald, W. I., Compston, A., Edan, G., Goodkin, D., Hartung, H.-P., Lublin, F. D., McFarland, H. F., et al. (2001). Recommended diagnostic criteria for multiple sclerosis: Guidelines from the international panel on the diagnosis of multiple sclerosis. *Annals of Neurology, 50*(1), 121–127.

McLaughlin, H. (2009). What's in a name: "client", "patient", "customer", "consumer", "expert by experience", "service user"—what's next? *British Journal of Social Work, 39*(6), 1101–1117.

Menzin, J., Caon, C., Nichols, C., White, L. A., Friedman, M., & Pill, M. W. (2012). Narrative review of the literature on adherence to disease-modifying therapies among patients with multiple sclerosis. *Journal of managed care pharmacy, 19*(1), 24–40.

Merleau-Ponty, M. (1962). Phenomenology of perception. *London: Routledge & Kegan Paul*.

Messina, M. J., Dalla Costa, G., Rodegher, M., Moiola, L., Colombo, B., Comi, G., & Martinelli, V. (2015). The communication of multiple sclerosis diagnosis: The patients' perspective. *Multiple sclerosis international, 2015*, doi: 10.1155/2015/353828.

Michel, L., Larochelle, C., & Prat, A. (2015). Update on treatments in multiple sclerosis. *La Presse Médicale*, *44*(4), e137–e151.

Miller, A. E., & Rhoades, R. W. (2012). Treatment of relapsing-remitting multiple sclerosis: current approaches and unmet needs. *Current opinion in neurology*, *25*, S4–S10.

Miller, C. E., & Jezewski, M. A. (2006). Relapsing MS patients' experiences with glatiramer acetate treatment: A phenomenological study. *Journal of Neuroscience Nursing*, *38*(1), 37–41.

Miller, C. E., Karpinski, M., & Jezewski, M. A. (2012). Relapsing-Remitting Multiple Sclerosis Patients' Experience with Natalizumab: A Phenomenological Investigation. *International journal of MS care*, *14*(1), 39–44.

Miller, C., & Jezewski, M. A. (2001). A Phenomenologic Assessment of Relapsing MS Patients' Experiences During Treatment With Interferon Beta-1a. *Journal of Neuroscience Nursing*, *33*(5), 240–244.

Miller, C. M. (1997). The lived experience of relapsing multiple sclerosis: A phenomenological study. *The Journal of Neuroscience Nursing*, *29*(5), 294–304.

Minis, M.-A. H., Satink, T., Kinébanian, A., Engels, J. A., Heerkens, Y. F., Engelen, B. G. van, & Sanden, M. W. Nijhuis-van der. (2014). How Persons with a Neuromuscular Disease Perceive Employment Participation: A Qualitative Study. *Journal of occupational rehabilitation*, *24*(1), 52–67.

Moran, D. (2002). *Introduction to Phenomenology*. London: Routledge.

Morgan, S., & Yoder, L. H. (2012). A concept analysis of person-centered care. *Journal of Holistic Nursing*, *30*(1), 6–15.

Morse, J. M. (2000). Determining sample size. *Qualitative health research*, *10*(1), 3–5.

Munir, F., Leka, S., & Griffiths, A. (2005). Dealing with self-management of chronic illness at work: Predictors for self-disclosure. *Social Science & Medicine*, *60*(6), 1397–1407.

Murray, S. J. (2007). Ethics at the scene of address: A conversation with Judith Butler. *Symposium,* 11(2)

415-445.

Murray, S. J. (2009). Aporia: Towards an ethic of critique. *Aporia, 1*(1), 8–14.

Murray, S. J. (2012). Phenomenology, ethics, and the crisis of the lived-body. *Nursing Philosophy, 13*(4), 289–294.

Murray, S. J., & Holmes, D. (2013). Toward a Critical Ethical Reflexivity: Phenomenology and Language in Maurice Merleau-Ponty. *Bioethics, 27*(6), 341–347.

Murray, S. J., & Holmes, D. (2014). Interpretive Phenomenological Analysis (IPA) and the Ethics of Body and Place: Critical Methodological Reflections. *Human Studies, 37*(1), 1–16.

Newman, J., & Tonkens, E. (2011). *Participation, responsibility and choice: Summoning the active citizen in western European welfare states*. Amsterdam: Amsterdam University Press.

Nortvedt, P., & Vosman, F. J. H. (2014). An Ethics of Care: New Perspectives, Both Theoretically and Empirically? *Nursing Ethics, 21*(7), 753–754.

Papathanasopoulos, P., Messinis, L., Lyros, E., Nikolakopoulou, A., Gourzoulidou, E., & Malefaki, S. (2008). Communicating the diagnosis of multiple sclerosis. *Journal of neurology, 255*(12), 1963–1969.

Papathanasopoulos, P., Nikolakopoulou, A., & Scolding, N. (2005). Disclosing the diagnosis of multiple sclerosis. *Journal of neurology, 252*(11), 1307–1309.

Patton, M. Q. (2005). *Qualitative research* (3rd ed.). Thousand Oaks, CA: Sage.

Payne, D., & McPherson, K. M. (2010). Becoming mothers. Multiple sclerosis and motherhood: A qualitative study. *Disability & Rehabilitation, 32*(8), 629–638.

Pfleger, C. C. H., Flachs, E. M., & Koch-Henriksen, N. (2010a). Social consequences of multiple sclerosis (1): Early pension and temporary unemployment-a historical prospective cohort study. *Multiple Sclerosis, 16*(1), 121–126.

Pfleger, C. C. H., Flachs, E. M., & Koch-Henriksen, N. (2010b). Social consequences of multiple sclerosis

(2): Divorce and separation: a historical prospective cohort study. *Multiple Sclerosis*, *16*(7), 878–882.

Philip, G. (2013). Extending the Analytical Lens': A Consideration of the Concepts of 'Care' and 'Intimacy' in Relation to Fathering After Separation or Divorce. *Sociological Research Online*, *18*(1), 15. [retrieved from http://www.socresonline.org.uk/18/1/15.html]

Pietkiewicz, I., & Smith, J. A. (2014). A practical guide to using Interpretative Phenomenological Analysis in qualitative research psychology. *Psychological Journal*, *20*(1), 7–14.

Polman, C. H., Reingold, S. C., Banwell, B., Clanet, M., Cohen, J. A., Filippi, M., Fujihara, K., et al. (2011). Diagnostic criteria for multiple sclerosis: 2010 revisions to the McDonald criteria. *Annals of neurology*, *69*(2), 292–302.

Prochaska, J. O., DiClemente, C. C., & Norcross, J. C. (1992). In search of how people change: Applications to addictive behaviors. *American Psychologist*, *47*(9), 1102-1114.

Rajagopalan, K., Brook, R. A., Beren, I. A., & Kleinman, N. L. (2010). Comparing costs and absences for multiple sclerosis among US employees: Pre- and post-treatment initiation. *Current Medical Research & Opinion*, *27*(1), 179–188.

Raphael, A., Hawkes, C., & Bernat, J. (2013). To tell or not to tell? Revealing the diagnosis in multiple sclerosis. *Multiple Sclerosis and Related Disorders*, *2*(3), 247–251.

Rolland, J. S. (2005). Cancer and the family: An integrative model. *Cancer*, *104*(S11), 2584–2595.

Sakellariou, D., Boniface, G., & Brown, P. (2013). Using Joint Interviews in a Narrative-Based Study on Illness Experiences. *Qualitative Health Research*, *23*(11), 1563–1570.

Samsi, K., Abley, C., Campbell, S., Keady, J., Manthorpe, J., Robinson, L., Watts, S., et al. (2014). Negotiating a Labyrinth: Experiences of assessment and diagnostic journey in cognitive impairment and dementia. *International journal of geriatric psychiatry*, *29*(1), 58–67.

Sander-Staudt, M. (2011). Care ethics. *Internet Encyclopedia of Philosophy*. [retrieved from http://www.iep.utm.edu/care-eth/]

Schmitz, H., Müllan, R. O., & Slaby, J. (2011). Emotions outside the box—the new phenomenology of feeling and corporeality. *Phenomenology and the Cognitive Sciences*, *10*(2), 241–259.

Schulman-Green, D., Jaser, S., Martin, F., Alonzo, A., Grey, M., McCorkle, R., Redeker, N. S., et al. (2012). Processes of Self-Management in Chronic Illness. *Journal of Nursing Scholarship*, *44*(2), 136–144.

Sencer, W. (1988). Suspicion of multiple sclerosis: To tell or not to tell? *Archives of Neurology*, *45*(4), 441–442.

Shields, C. G., Finley, M. A., Chawla, N., & others. (2012). Couple and family interventions in health problems. *Journal of marital and family therapy*, *38*(1), 265–280.

Sholl, J. (2015). Putting phenomenology in its place: Some limits of a phenomenology of medicine. *Theoretical medicine and bioethics*, *36*(6), 391–410.

Smith, J. A. (1996). Beyond the divide between cognition and discourse: Using interpretative phenomenological analysis in health psychology. *Psychology and health*, *11*(2), 261–271.

Smith, J. A., Flowers, P., & Larkin, M. (2009). *Interpretative Phenomenological Analysis: Theory, Method and Research*. Los Angeles, CA: SAGE Publications.

Springer, R. A. (2011). Pharmaceutical Industry discursives and the marketization of nursing work: a case example. *Nursing Philosophy*, *12*, 214-228.

Stahl, D. (2013). Living into the imagined body: how the diagnostic image confronts the lived body. *Medical Humanities*, *39*, 53-58. doi:10.1136/medhum-2012-010286.

Solari, A., Acquarone, N., Pucci, E., Martinelli, V., Marrosu, M., Trojano, M., Borreani, C., et al. (2007). Communicating the diagnosis of multiple sclerosis-a qualitative study. *Multiple Sclerosis*, *13*(6), 763–769.

Sweetland, J., Howse, E., & Playford, E. D. (2012). A systematic review of research undertaken in vocational rehabilitation for people with multiple sclerosis. *Disability and Rehabilitation*, *34*(24),

2031–2038.

Sweetland, J., Riazi, A., Cano, S. J., & Playford, E. D. (2007). Vocational rehabilitation services for people with multiple sclerosis: what patients want from clinicians and employers. *Multiple Scleroris*, *13*(9), 1183–1189.

Ten Have, H. (1995). The anthropological tradition in the philosophy of medicine. *Theoretical medicine*, *16*(1), 3–14.

Ten Have, H., & Gordijn, B. (2014). The significance of relatedness in healthcare. *Medicine, health care, and philosophy*, *17*(2), 169.

Tiedtke, C., Rijk, A. de, Donceel, P., Christiaens, M.-R., & Casterlé, B. D. de. (2012). Survived but feeling vulnerable and insecure: A qualitative study of the mental preparation for RTW after breast cancer treatment. *BMC Public Health*, *12*(1), 538–550.

Todres, L., Galvin, K. T., & Dahlberg, K. (2014). "Caring for insiderness": Phenomenologically informed in-

sights that can guide practice. *International journal of qualitative studies on health and well-being*, *9*, doi: 10.3402/qhw.v9.21421.

Tong, A., Sainsbury, P., & Craig, J. (2007). Consolidated criteria for reporting qualitative research (COREQ): A 32-item checklist for interviews and focus groups. *International Journal for Quality in Health Care*, *19*(6), 349–357.

Toombs, S. K. (1988). Illness and the paradigm of lived body. *Theoretical medicine*, *9*(2), 201–226.

Toombs, S. K. (1995). The Lived Experience of Disability. *Human Studies*, *18*(1), 9–24.

Toombs, S. K. (2001). The role of empathy in clinical practice. *Journal of Consciousness Studies*, *8*(5-7), 247–258.

Toombs, S. K. (2004). 'Is she experiencing any pain?': Disability and the physician-patient relationship.

Internal Medicine Journal, *34*(11), 645–647.

Tronto, J. C. (1993). *Moral boundaries: A political argument for an ethic of care*. New York, N.Y.: Routlegde.

Van Nes, F., Abma, T., Jonsson, H., & Deeg, D. (2010). Language differences in qualitative research: Is meaning lost in translation? *European journal of ageing*, *7*(4), 313–316.

Varekamp, I., Heutink, A., Landman, S., Koning, C. E., Vries, G. de, & Dijk, F. J. van (2009). Facilitating empowerment in employees with chronic disease: qualitative analysis of the process of change. *Journal of occupational rehabilitation*, *19*(4), 398–408.

Visser, L., & Zande, A. van der (2011). Reasons patients give to use or not to use immunomodulating agents for multiple sclerosis. *European Journal of Neurology*, *18*(11), 1343–1349.

Vosman, F. J. H., & Baart, A. (2009). Being witness to the lives of the very old. *Journal of Social Intervention: Theory and Practice*, *17*(3), 21–32.

Vossen, E., & Gestel, N. van (2015). The activation logic in national sickness absence policies: Comparing the Netherlands, Denmark and Ireland. *European Journal of Industrial Relations*, *21*(2), 165–80.

Waksler, F. C. (2001). Medicine and the phenomenological method. *Handbook of phenomenology and medicine* (pp. 67–86). Dordecht: Springer.

Wisner, A. (1972). Diagnosis in ergonomics: The choice of operating models in field research. *Ergonomics, 15*(6) 601-620.

Wisner, A., Veil, C., & Dejours, C. (1985). Psychopathologie du travail. *Paris: Entreprise Moderne d'Edition*, 102–104.

Yadav, V., Bever, C., Bowen, J., Bowling, A., Weinstock-Guttman, B., Cameron, M., Bourdette, D., et al. (2014). Summary of evidence-based guideline: Complementary and alternative medicine in multiple sclerosis Report of the Guideline Development Subcommittee of the American Academy of Neurology. *Neurology*, *82*(12), 1083–1092.

Ziemssen, T., Hoffman, J., Apfel, R., & Kern, S. (2008). Effects of glatiramer acetate on fatigue and days of absence from work in first-time treated relapsing-remitting multiple sclerosis. *Health an Quality*

of Life Outcomes, 6(67), 67–72.

Summary

Professional loving care is a moral approach to professional healthcare, drawing on ethic of care and presence theory. Ethic of care is a moral theory that maintains the moral significance of relationships and dependencies in human life. It was first developed by Gilligan and Noddings in the eighties of the previous century. Ten years later, the seminal book "Moral Boundaries" of Tronto sparked the interest of Dutch and Flemish ethicists, including Van Heijst, Baart, Grypdonk and Gastmans, in ethic of care. In "Moral Boundaries", Tronto explores ethic of care as a political theory. Her work signalled a new phase in the development of ethic of care worldwide. Typically for the Dutch and Flemish reception of this phase is that it often joins the advancement of moral and political theory with insights from qualitative research. One idea behind this combination is that insight in the lived experiences of patients can serve as an heuristic tool for health care professionals and those involved in ethical deliberation. With qualitative research, they can uncover the complexity and richness of the dependencies and relationships that frame the world in which patients live their lives. Insight in complexity and richness helps them to attune their relationships closer to the perspectives of patients. A second argument for the association of ethical reflection with empirical research is that empirical groundedness amplifies and advances the development of moral theory.

In this study, we explore lived experiences of 10 people recently (<2 years) diagnosed with relapsing remitting multiple sclerosis (MS). We invited these people, two men and eight women, aged between 27 and 51 years, to share lived experiences of illness and daily life. We did this by offering them an occasion to create, in the environment of their own homes and in front of another person (a researcher), a spoken account of how lived illness and life originally presented themselves to them and affected them as persons. Although we encouraged the participants to speak freely, we also employed a topic list to add a certain degree of structure to the encounters. This topic list addressed diagnosis, personal situation, care and work. All participants indeed expanded on these topics. Also they added to these topics a forth one, evolving around the (non) use of disease modifying treatment (drugs). In the main section of this study, "lived experiences", we reconstruct the "voice of experience" (of illness and daily life) and untangle it from "the voice of medicine". In this "voice", strongly present in, and sometime even dominating the accounts, spoken language is a tool to communicate an objectivised message about disease. But proper to the "voice of experience" is language understood as an embodied capacity that allows speakers to create and share unique meanings and personal perspectives, including personal experiences on suffering and pain.

In the **first chapter,** we explore lived experiences evolving around the process of MS diagnoses. Within the selection of participants, perceptions of the process of diagnosis greatly varied. For some, the diagnosis meant the conclusion of years of living with unexplained physical complaints and numerous medical investigations by physicians from various medical specialties. But for others, the occurrence of physical complaints (including reduced sight, wobbly limbs and numbness) was so quickly followed by the finding of the proper diagnosis that the two were experienced as aspects of one single event. For all participants, the day of the disclosure of the (provisional) diagnosis was unforgettable. Most participants described intensified awareness of persons, spaces (especially the MRI scanner), atmospheres, conversations and one's own body and mind before, during and after the disclosure of the diagnosis. Some lived phenomena presented themselves with a vibrant relational twist. For some participants the time of uncertainty between provisional and definitive diagnosis was a time to align closer with parents or partner. Others maintained how important it was for them that the physician that disclosed the diagnosis was able to relate to their feelings and emotions at that moment. We conclude the chapter with the observation that despite the advent of patient centred care, attention for the perspective of the patient in directives for good medical care in MS is still marginal.

In the **second chapter,** we explore lived experiences evolving around the use of disease modifying therapies (DMT) in MS. Medial directives instruct physicians to advise patients to start the use of DMT soon after the establishment of the diagnosis. All ten participants of our study were advised to start DMT. Seven of them used medication at the time of the interview. Six of them used injectable medication (*interferon beta 1a* or *glatiramer acetate*) and one a drug in tablet form (*fingolimod*). Most (but not all) participants told that initially they received the advice to start DMT with feelings of restraint and reluctance. These feelings were described with spatial and temporal metaphors like "being not yet ready to start", "crossing a barrier to start" and "illness comes too close". The feelings of users and non-users referred to the mode of administration (injections or tablets), the substance itself as well as the (high) frequency of administration. Some users of DMT gave detailed descriptions of the application of tools for administration (injection pens) at their own bodies while others highlighted the use of DMT as a way to preserve hope and to influence the course of MS. Gaining trust to start appeared to be important for users of DMT and some participants maintained how the support of others (medical professionals and close intimates) had been vital to gain and preserve that trust. We conclude the chapter with the observation that starting DMT means for patients a lot more than adherence to a directive. It would be a good idea for physicians to take this into account when advising patients to start DMT.

In the **third chapter,** we zoom in at the family as an important horizon or background for lived experiences of illness and daily life. For each of the participants this horizon looked different. For some of them this horizon lied at some distance in front of them. It was felt how MS blurred future perspectives at finding a partner, raising children and even at control over how to be remembered as a parent in old age or after decease. Other participants experienced gradations in to what extent they felt MS to be an element of the family as a shared horizon for living. They sometimes felt a tension between the wish to keep MS (fatigue and reduced mobility) with themselves and the wish to release it to become part of daily living with intimates. For some participants, the lived dynamics of hiding and showing MS was aligned with a sense of guilt with regard to children, depended on their care, and with a struggle to accept help from parents or partner. The findings in the third chapter complicate the romantic picture in ethic of care of becoming of a recipient of care (within the horizon of family life) as the unfolding of a new opportunity to live a moral life. For people recently diagnosed with MS, need for help is often a sad thing and related with grief over lost dreams and physical capacities. Receiving help is not experienced as a new mode for a good life. But even so the findings complicate also romantic tropes found elsewhere of the family as a straightforward resource for care.

In the **fourth chapter,** we present experiences lived within social structures wherein people do paid work. Within the selection of participants, perceptions of and within such structures greatly varied. The two youngest participants hadn't even started their career at the moment of the interview. For them paid work was something that they anticipated rather than lived. The nature of their disease made one participant to feel concerned about the likelihood of a career shorter than previously planned. Another felt urged by MS to aim at an alternative career path, better suited for an episodic and progressive disease. Also the five participants that already (or still) had a job, worried about the future. The possibility of making a move to another employer or even toward another profession was no longer felt. Some participants anticipated reduction of working hours or struggled with mangers to adapt physical and organisational conditions of their job to the demands of their disease. For three participants, paid work definitively already had become an issue of the past. One participant understood the present situation of living from a social benefit as preferable above a previously experienced intricate situation of working in a regular job while having an irregular disease. But for the two others, the view towards the past dominated their perspective. Memories about a terminated career sparked feelings of sadness and grief. Very few theories diverge from the dominant functionalist and psychological approaches to work. Very few theories hence address work as a perspectival and relational issue. In the final section of the chapter, we bring up the scare theories that address work as such and do we argue for the need for more research in this area.

In the **final section**, the **discussion,** we uphold the idea that, against a background of ethic of care, attention to the "voice of experience" of patients is a native and perhaps even the defining aspect of morally significant relationships between professional providers of MS care and their patients. Phenomenology remains an obvious candidate to conceive and investigate this voice, in spite of two recent objections against phenomenology as a method for clarification of issues in medicine. This study has yielded a taste of how the voice of experience of people recently diagnosed with MS sounds like. Part of this this yield was a view at how people with a serious and chronic disease live relationships. Lived loss of control seems to be a persistent aspect. People have to start relationships with unfamiliar medical professionals. Disease obstructs efforts to retain jobs and hence contacts with colleagues. The lived dynamics of hiding and showing MS within the horizon of family life shows how disease unsettles relationships with children, partner and parents. But we observed sometimes also a second and more uplifting aspect in lived relationships. The challenge to start with lifelong use of drugs motivated some participants to reach out for moral and practical support. Participants perceived how the uncertainty during the testing for MS boosted loving commitment from family, friends and colleagues.

Ethic of care says that there is moral significance in relationships and dependencies. In this study, relationships and dependencies surfaced occasionally as elements in lived experiences. Broadly speaking these relationships and dependencies involved mostly in one way or another loss of control. But at some occasions they also meant the discovery of true commitment and concern from others. We hesitate to qualify these occasions as instances in which moral significance of relationships showed itself. We think that "moral significance" is a fundamental category that people sometimes use to signify something as deeply valuable and human. But we don't feel that participants felt that strong about the occasions at which they experienced concern and love. However we suggest that things – including an empirical ethic of care in MS - can be conceived in degrees of intensity. Out of wonder and amazement about loyalty and friendship during hard times, might gradually grow new insight. This insight may mean that also living in a increasing state of dependency from others, can account for a full human life. Continued research in lived experiences of MS and other conditions is necessary to enhance the outlook of our study at how the beginning and initial development of such insights actually can look like.

Samenvatting

Menslievende zorg is een morele benadering van professionele gezondheidszorg waarvan de theoretische achtergrond gevormd wordt door zorgethiek en de presentietheorie. Zorgethiek is een theorie die relaties en afhankelijkheid ziet als mogelijkheden voor moreel leven. De theorie werd ontworpen door Gilligan en Noddings in de jaren tachtig van de vorige eeuw. Een decennium later arriveerde zorgethiek, via het boek "Moral Bounderies" van zorgethica Tronto, in het werk van Vlaamse en Nederlandse ethici, waaronder Van Heijst, Grypdonk en Gastmans. Tronto was de eerste die zorgethiek uitwerkte tot een politieke theorie. Haar boek vormde wereldwijd het begin van een nieuwe fase in de ontwikkeling van zorgethiek. Kenmerkend voor de Vlaamse en Nederlandse receptie van zorgethiek is dat ze morele en politieke reflectie combineert met het doen van kwalitatief onderzoek. Een eerste argument voor deze combinatie is dat inzicht in geleefde ervaringen een hulpmiddel is voor zorgverleners en ethici voor het ontwikkelen van goede zorg. Met kwalitatief onderzoek kan zicht worden gekregen op de rijkdom en de complexiteit van de relaties en afhankelijkheden. Deze vormen een belangrijk element van de leefwereld van patiënten en zorgverleners. Inzicht in verscheidenheid en complexiteit kan zorgverleners en zorgethici helpen zorg beter af te stemmen op de behoeften en zienswijzen van patiënten. Een tweede argument voor het combineren van morele reflectie met kwalitatief onderzoek is dat empirische fundering de ontwikkeling van zorgethiek als morele theorie voedt en versterkt.

In dit proefschrift onderzoek ik de geleefde ervaringen van een groep van tien personen met een recente (< 2 jaar) diagnose multiple sclerose (MS) van *relapsing-remitting* type. Deze groep, bestaande uit twee mannen en acht vrouwen in de leeftijd van 27 tot 51 jaar, werd uitgenodigd om mij en mijn medeonderzoekers deelgenoot te maken van hun ervaringen met ziekte en dagelijks leven. De werkvorm die we daarvoor aanboden, bestond uit een interview met een onderzoeker bij de participant thuis, op een door de participant gekozen moment. De gesprekken met de participanten hadden een open karakter. Tegelijkertijd maakte ik en de andere twee interviewers gebruik van een lijst met vier onderwerpen om aan de gesprekken een zekere mate van structuur te geven. Deze onderwerpen waren diagnose, persoonlijke situatie, zorg, en werk.

Alle participanten gingen uitgebreid in op deze onderwerpen. Tegelijkertijd bleek uit de interviews dat de participanten nog een vijfde onderwerp van belang vonden; het al dan niet gebruiken van medicijnen. In het middendeel van dit proefschrift, getiteld "lived experiences" (geleefde ervaringen), ontrafel ik uit de interviews de stem van geleefde ervaringen (subjectieve benadering van ziekte) en onderscheid ik die stem van de stem van de geneeskunde (objectieve benadering van ziekte). De stem van de geneeskunde was in elk interview pregnant aanwezig. Daarnaast echter klinkt ook de stem van de ervaring. Deze stem opent zicht op hoe participanten, vanuit hun eigen perspectief, ziekte en zorg waarnemen en betekenis geven.

In **hoofdstuk een** onderzoek ik geleefde ervaringen rondom het vaststellen van de diagnose MS. Vervolgens betrek ik deze ervaringen op de vraag naar de ontwikkeling van persoonsgerichte patiëntenzorg. Zelfs binnen de betrekkelijk kleine groep participanten verschilden de waarnemingen van het proces van het vaststellen van de diagnose in hoge mate. Voor sommigen betekende het vaststellen van de diagnose de afronding van jaren leven met onverklaarbare klachten en talloze onderzoeken bij meerdere medisch specialisten. Voor anderen daarentegen volgende op het voelen van de eerste klachten (waaronder verminderd zicht en zwalkende of dove ledematen) al heel snel de juiste diagnose, waardoor het voelen van de klachten en het vinden van de diagnose werden ervaren als twee onderdelen van dezelfde gebeurtenis. Alle participanten gaven aan dat ze de dag waarop ze de diagnose te horen kregen nooit meer zouden vergeten. De meeste participanten beschreven rondom het vaststellen van de diagnose een verscherpte waarneming van personen, ruimten (in het bijzonder de MRI scanner), sfeer, gesprekken, het eigen lijf, de eigen gedachtenstroom. In enkele geleefde ervaringen kwam een prominente plaats voor relationaliteit aan het licht. Zo betekende voor sommigen de onzekere tijd tussen de voorlopige en de definitieve diagnose verdieping van de relaties met ouders of partner. Anderen benadrukten hoe belangrijk het voor hen was geweest dat op het moment van het vertellen van de diagnose de dokter in staat was om rekening te houden met de emoties die op dat moment speelden. Ik besluit het hoofdstuk met de vaststelling dat, ondanks de opkomende aandacht voor het belang van persoonsgerichte patiëntenzorg, in richtlijnen en reflecties over goede MS zorg, het patiëntenperspectief nog steeds een onderbelicht thema is.

In **hoofdstuk twee** onderzoek ik geleefde ervaringen met betrekking tot het gebruik van ziekte remmende medicijnen voor MS. Richtlijnen adviseren dokters om hun patiënten snel na de diagnose te laten starten met zulke medicijnen. Alle participanten van mijn promotieonderzoek hadden van hun arts het advies gekregen om te beginnen met ziekteremmers. Zeven van hen gebruikten ook daadwerkelijk medicatie op het moment dat ze geïnterviewd werden. Zes gebruikers injecteerden hun medicatie (*interferon beta 1a* of *glatiramer acetate*) en één gebruikte een tablet (*fingolimod*). De meeste (maar niet alle) participanten gaven aan dat zij het advies om te starten met medicatie gereserveerdheid hadden ontvangen. Hun aarzelingen drukten ze uit met ruimtelijke en temporele metaforen als "er nog niet klaar voor zijn", "een drempel over moeten", en "de ziekte komt (te) dichtbij". De geleefde ervaringen van gebruikers en niet-gebruikers hadden betrekking op de wijze van toediening (met injecties of door tabletten), de samenstelling van de medicatie, en de frequentie van toediening. Sommige gebruikers gaven gedetailleerde beschrijvingen het gebruik van hulpmiddelen voor toediening (vooral wanneer ze injectiespuiten gebruikten). Anderen benadrukten hoe het gebruik van medicijnen voor hen een manier was om hoop te houden en het verloop van hun ziekte te beïnvloeden. Alle gebruikers ervoeren dat het hen moeite had gekost om moed te verzamelen om te beginnen en door te zetten. Ze merkten op hoe belangrijk de steun van anderen (medische professionals en familieleden en vrienden) daarin geweest was. Ik sluit het hoofdstuk af met de observatie dat het starten van het gebruik van ziekte remmende medicatie voor patiënten veel méér betekent dan enkel het zich confirmeren aan de medische richtlijn. Het is aan te bevelen dat dokters met dit surplus aan betekenis rekening houden, wanneer zij het opstarten van MS medicatie met hun patiënten bespreken.

In **hoofdstuk drie** zoom ik in op de familie als een belangrijke sociale structuur waarin ziekte en dagelijks leven ervaren worden. De vormgeving van deze structuur en het persoonlijk perspectief erop verschilden van participant tot participant. Sommigen merkten dat ze vooral met de toekomst bezig waren. Ze vreesden dat hun ziekte een spelbreker zou worden bij het vinden van een levensgezel, bij het opvoeden van nakomelingen en bij de wijze waarop hun kinderen zich later hun jeugd met een zieke ouder zouden herinneren. Andere participanten ervoeren gradaties in de mate waarin hun ziekte deelden met het familieverband waarin zij leefden. Deze participanten ervoeren een spanning tussen de wens om de gevolgen van hun ziekte (vermoeidheid en verminderde mobiliteit) te verhullen en de wens juist met naasten de ziekte en het verdriet daarover te delen. Voor sommige participanten hing de spanning tussen verhullen en delen samen met schuldgevoel richting kinderen, die van hun zorg afhankelijk waren, of met een worsteling om mantelzorg te aanvaarden van partner of ouders. Het beeld van zorg dat oprijst uit het derde hoofdstuk compliceert het soms idyllische beeld in zorgethiek van zorgrelaties van families als moreel betekenisvolle verbanden waarop iemand terug kan vallen in geval van ziek en afhankelijk worden. Voor de participanten was het afhankelijk worden van zorg dikwijls een verdrietige gebeurtenis die verbonden was met rouw over gebroken toekomstverwachtingen en verminderde lichamelijke conditie. De door ziekte opkomende zorgrelaties werden niet altijd ervaren als een alternatieve mogelijkheid voor een waardevol leven, wat een kerngedachte van de zorgethiek is. De geleefde ervaringen die in dit hoofdstuk worden gesproken, nuanceren het beeld van familie als een ongecompliceerde basis om op terug te vallen als er zorg nodig is. Ziekte wordt ook ervaren als bedreiging voor de familie waarin de ziekte geleefd wordt.

In **hoofdstuk vier** richt ik mijn aandacht op betaald werk als een sociale structuur waarin ziekte geleefd wordt. Net als in het vorige hoofdstuk verschilde de vormgeving van deze structuur en het persoonlijk perspectief erop van participant tot participant. Voor de jongste twee deelnemers was een loopbaan iets dat nog voor hen lag. Een van hen maakte zich zorgen over de duur van haar loopbaan. Ze voorzag dat die korter gaan zou gaan duren dan ze voorheen dacht. De andere participant voldoende zich door haar diagnose gedwongen na te denken over een alternatieve loopbaan die beter te combineren zou zijn met haar ziekte. De vier participanten die een baan hadden op het moment van het interview maakten zich zorgen over de toekomst. Ze voelden zich door hun ziekte niet vrij om te wisselen van werkgever of van professie. Een aantal van hen overwoog minder te gaan werken of ervoer spanningen met leidinggevenden over het aanpassen van de werkplek en het verminderen van werkuren en werkbelasting. Voor drie participanten was werk een zaak geworden die ze reeds achter zich hadden gelaten. Een van hen vond dat hij in een leven met de zekerheid van een sociale uitkering beter af was dan toen hij nog werkte. Toen moest hij verwachtingen omtrent hem als een betrouwbare werknemer zien te combineren met een onvoorspelbare, moeilijk te controleren ziekte. De andere twee echter, hoewel inmiddels zonder baan, hadden hun werkzame verleden gevoelsmatig *niet* achter zich gelaten. Het zich herinneren van hun vroegtijdig afgebroken loopbaan vervulde hen met spijt en verdriet. In theorieën over werk hebben psychologiserende en functionalistische benaderingen de overhand. Voor werk als relationeel en subjectief ervaren fenomeen is nauwelijks aandacht. Op het einde van dit hoofdstuk bespreken ik enkele theorieën die werk als zodanig analyseren en benadruk ik dat meer onderzoek naar werk als relationeel en subjectief fenomeen nodig is.

In de **discussie** die dit proefschrift afsluit, betoog ik dat, vanuit de zorgethische achtergrond van dit proefschrift, aandacht voor de stem van ervaring door zorgverleners waarschijnlijk een kernelement is van menslievende zorg voor mensen met MS. Ondanks de recente tegenwerpingen van twee auteurs tegen fenomenologie als methode voor de opheldering van medische vraagstukken, zijn er goede redenen om deze benadering te blijven zien als een waardevol instrument voor het waarnemen en onderzoeken van de stem van ervaring. De opbrengst van dit proefschrift is een proeve van de klank van geleefde ervaringen van mensen met een recente diagnose MS. Een onderdeel van die opbrengst was inzicht in hoe mensen met een ernstige chronische aandoening als MS relaties ervaren. Geleefd verlies van controle binnen relaties is een aspect dat dikwijls voortdurend terugkwam in de interviews. Mensen moeten relaties aanknopen met nieuwe en onbekende zorgverleners. Ziekte problematiseert het vasthouden van betaald werk en het contact met collega's. De geleefde dynamiek van het verhullen en delen van MS binnen familieverband liet zien hoe ziekte relaties met kinderen, partner en ouders verandert. Een aantal keren echter vonden we ook een tweede en gelukkiger aspect van geleefde relaties van mensen met MS. De uitdaging om te starten met het chronisch gebruik van medicijnen motiveerde enkele participanten om praktische en morele steun te zoeken. Andere participanten ontdekten hoe zij in onzekere periode rondom het stellen van de diagnose konden rekenen op de liefdevolle betrokkenheid van familie, vrienden en collega's.

Zorgethiek stelt dat afhankelijkheid en relaties een intrinsieke morele waarden hebben. In dit proefschrift dienden afhankelijkheid en relaties zo nu en dan zich aan als onderdelen van geleefde ervaringen. Over het algemeen betekende het ontstaan zorgrelaties en afhankelijkheid voor de participanten het op een of andere wijze verliezen van regie. Een enkele keer echter impliceerde het ontstaan van afhankelijkheid van zorg inderdaad het ontstaan van de moreel betekenisvolle relaties en afhankelijkheid waarom het in de zorgethiek draait.

Acknowledgements

I want to express thanks to the two supervisors of my dissertation, prof. dr. Frans J. H. Vosman and prof. dr. Leo H. Visser. I during my voluntary commitment as an editor (2004-2011) for *Tijdschrift Geestelijke Verzorging*, a Dutch journal for professional spiritual and pastoral care, I had become aware of dr. Vosman due to his thoughtful contributions and because of his sympathy for the work of health care chaplains. Dr. Vosman and I learned that we shared critical insights about care, subjectivity and sense making and from this point a joint research project emerged. Dr. Vosman has maintained during his supervision always a stimulating atmosphere of encouragement and friendship, also when organizational changes and illness made his work more difficult to do. Also the supervision of dr. Visser has been vital. He enabled my project to become empirical due to its association with the neurology department of the Elisabeth-TweeSteden Ziekenhuis. He facilitated the donation of a research grant by the Dutch National MS Foundation, Maassluis. Also in the advanced stages of the project he remained a critical, committed and very practical commentator of my work. Dr. Gert Olthuis has contributed significantly to the development of the research design and was a valuable member of the four member team that completed the initial analysis of the audio transcriptions of the interviews. His humour and "hands on" mentality made working together pleasing and inspiring. Drs. Daphne Frijlink MD interviewed three participants and transcribed the related audio files. Stan van Zon MA has assisted me very helpfully as copy editor.

www.ingramcontent.com/pod-product-compliance
Lightning Source LLC
Chambersburg PA
CBHW041444210326
41599CB00004B/131